Bilingual Vocabulary for the Medical Profession

Vocabulario bilingüe para la profesión médica

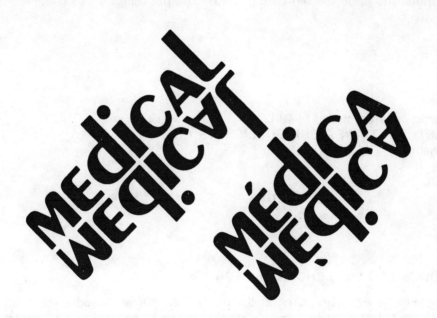

Ralph Escandón,
Pacific Union College,
Angwin, California

V69 **SOUTH-WESTERN PUBLISHING CO.**

CINCINNATI   WEST CHICAGO, ILL.   DALLAS   PELHAM MANOR, N.Y.   PALO ALTO, CALIF.

ISBN: 0-538-22690-0
Library of Congress Catalog Card Number 81-52249
1 2 3 4 5 6 7 8 9 0 Ki 1 0 9 8 7 6 5 4 3 2
Impreso en los Estados Unidos de América
(Printed in the United States of America)

CONTENTS / CONTENIDO

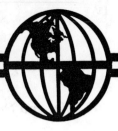

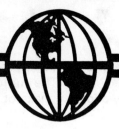

Guide to English and Spanish Pronunciation — Guía de pronunciación española e inglesa

The English alphabet has 26 letters.

a, b, c, d, e, f, g, h, i, j, k, l, m, n, o, p, q, r, s, t, u, v, w, x, y, z

El alfabeto del inglés tiene 26 letras.

Vowel Sounds, Simple: Model Words

beet, chief, queen, seed
bit, mill, quit
bait, quaint, rate, way
bet, men, question, well
burr, her, quirk
bud, mother, rut

Vocales sencillas: palabras modelo

boot, fruit, shoe, who
bull, foot, took
boat, hoe, Ho!, quote, show, wrote
bottle, quash
bond, quandary, yonder

Vowel Sounds, Compound (diphthongs): Model Words

height, hyper, light, quite
boy, choice, groin, royal

Vocales compuestas (diptongos): palabras modelo

beautiful, mule, union
about, cow, Howdy!

Consonant Sounds: Model Words

pipe
bumble
tatter
dud
kicked
gagged
fluff
revive
thing, monolith
that, rather
secede
dazzles, raises, zones
shall, Fischer, sure

Consonantes: palabras modelo

azure, measure
chin, watch
edge, just, urge
ma'am
nine
sink
thing
loll
roar
hat, who
yo-yo
fix (ks)
exaggerate (gz)

In some cases, other spelling combinations may also be used to represent these sounds.

En algunos casos, otras combinaciones de letras también pueden ser empleadas para representar estos sonidos.

Students: When you are in doubt about the pronunciation of a word in English or Spanish, ask your instructor to pronounce the **model words** that contain the sounds that make up that word.

Al estudiante: Si tiene alguna duda acerca de cómo debe ser pronunciada una palabra o del inglés o del español, pídale al profesor que pronuncie las **palabras modelo** que contengan los sonidos que integran esa palabra.

The Spanish alphabet can include as many as 29 letters. The multiple pronunciation of **rr**, in addition, make of it a separate sound.

El alfabeto del español puede abarcar hasta 29 letras. También hay que tener en cuenta la pronunciación múltiple de la **doble r,** lo cual hace de ella un sonido aparte.

a, b, c, ch, d, e, f, g, h, i, j, k, l, ll, m, n, ñ, o, p, q, r, (rr), s, t, u, v, w, x, y, z

Vowel Sounds, simple: Model Words

abarcar
El merecerá
A él réntenle
insistir

Vocales sencillas: palabras modelo

ronroneo
los ojos
cucurucho

Vowel Sounds, Compound (diphthongs): Model Words

amainar, vaina, ¡Caray!
¡Albricias!, ajiaco
aumentar, pauta
Juan, cualitativo
pleito, veleidad, carey
tiene, sentimiento
pleuresía, reuma

Vocales compuestas (diptongos): palabras modelo

huevo, ahuecar
ciudad, piune
cuidado, whiskey
hoy, Moisés, prohibido
miope, propio
promiscuo, cuota

Consonant Sounds: Model Words (Most common Spanish-American pronunciation)

cavaba, la boba, el vivo, el Wolframio
convenio, ¡caramba!, ¡Ven!, ¡Beba!
casco, kilo, quiere, Querétaro
caldo, candente, ¡Dámelo!
chasco, muchacho
la duda, ardid
fofo, énfasis
¡Está gagá!, algo, la guerra
¡Póngalo!, ¡Ganemos!
hijo, desahucio
jauja, Jujuy, giba, agente
alelado, luna

Consonantes: palabras modelo (pronunciación hispanoamericana más común)

llama, calle, ya, ayo, hiena
amamantar, momento
nonada, cándido, llavín
ñame, caño
popular, campo
aro, arará, apuntar
¡Ríense!, carro, enredo, arrulla
zonzo, suceso, ácido
matute, tirantes
extra (gs)
laxo (ks)

Students: When you are in doubt about the pronunciation of a word in English or Spanish, ask your instructor to pronounce the **model words** that contain the sounds that make up that word.

Al estudiante: Si tiene alguna duda acerca de cómo debe ser pronunciada una palabra o del inglés o del español, pídale al instructor que pronuncie las **palabras modelo** que contengan los sonidos que integren esa palabra.

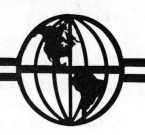

Spanish is the second most important language in the world, and the fourth in the number of people who speak it. The most widespread language in the world is English, followed by Spanish. English, the language of Shakespeare, and Spanish, known as the language of Cervantes, together dominate the Western Hemisphere. The influence of Spanish is felt in most of the countries of the three Americas, from the United States to Cape Horn, with some exceptions, such as Brazil, the Guianas, and a few Caribbean islands. Spanish is also spoken in Spain, and is well known in some European countries. Its influence extends from North Africa to the Philippines, where some of the older generations still speak it.

Of the thirteen most important languages in the world, seven of them (English, Spanish, French, Portuguese, Italian, German, and Russian) are of European origin, while the other six are of Asiatic stock. Spanish, along with French, Portuguese, Italian, Catalonian, and Rumanian, comprise the Romance branch, which derives from Vulgar Latin.

Bilingual Vocabulary for the Medical Profession is part of a series of bilingual books designed to meet the multiple needs of true bilingual (Spanish-English) training. The series includes books by other authors: **Bilingual Business Grammar, Personal Business, Skills for the Business World, Bilingual Business Careers, Be Bilingual I and II, Skills for Bilingual Legal Personnel, Spanish-English Legal Terminology, Topics for Business English for Spanish Speaking Students,** and others.

This book is an elementary treatise of Spanish-English, geared to the health field and

El español es el segundo idioma más importante en el mundo de hoy, y ocupa el cuarto lugar con relación al número de personas que lo hablan. Después del inglés, el español es el idioma más popular. La lengua de Cervantes se habla en casi todo el Hemisferio Occidental, desde los Estados Unidos de América hasta el Cabo de Hornos, con la sola excepción del Brazil, las Guayanas y unas pocas islas del Caribe. También se habla en España y se le conoce bien en algunos países europeos. Su influencia se extiende hasta el Africa del Norte y las Islas Filipinas, en donde algunas personas todavía lo hablan.

De los trece idiomas más importantes del mundo de hoy, siete de ellos (inglés, español, francés, portugués, italiano, alemán y ruso) tienen procedencia europea; mientras que los otros seis tienen sus orígenes en las lenguas asiáticas. El español, juntamente con el francés, el portugués, el italiano, el catalán y el rumano constituyen las lenguas romances, las cuales se originaron del latín vulgar.

Este texto, **Vocabulario bilingüe para la profesión médica** es parte de una serie de libros destinados a proveer los diversos elementos que componen una completa preparación bilingüe (español-inglés). La serie incluye varios libros, escritos por diversos autores, tales como: **Gramática comercial bilingüe, Asuntos personales, Conocimientos para el mundo del comercio, Carreras comerciales bilingües, Sea bilingüe I y II, Técnicas para el personal bilingüe en el área legal, Terminología español-inglés en el área legal, Temas para inglés comercial para estudiantes de habla hispana,** y otros más.

El presente texto es un tratado elemental de español-inglés, con un enfoque hacia el campo

intended to be useful to doctors, nurses, hospital personnel and medical secretaries.

To make it practical, as well as useful, some Spanish-English grammar has been included together with the conversations, bilingual projects, readings, and exercises related to the medical profession.

The main purpose of this textbook is to inspire students to learn both languages while getting acquainted with medical terminology in Spanish-English. At the end of the book there is a selected vocabulary of many medically-related terms.

Bilingual Vocabulary for the Medical Profession is divided into lessons by topic. The main components of each lesson are: vocabularies, conversations, grammatical hints, additional pertinent information, a bilingual project (preparatory exercise or transcription), and exercises. The student is asked to turn to the Index at the end of the book for a more detailed reference guide.

I hope, dear student, that at the end of this course you will not only have learned vocabulary and medical expressions, but will also be able to speak these beautiful languages and understand something of the varied cultural heritages involved.

médico. El libro se preparó con el propósito de rendir un servicio a médicos, enfermeras, personal administrativo de hospital, secretarias de médicos y demás personal bilingüe en el campo de la medicina. Con este fin en mente, se han incluido algunas reglas gramaticales relacionadas con las conversaciones, lecturas, proyectos bilingües y ejercicios en cada lección.

El propósito primordial de este libro es inspirar a los estudiantes para que se dediquen al aprendizaje de ambos idiomas, al mismo tiempo que adquieren una preparación bilingüe específica del campo médico. Al final del libro se presenta un vocabulario selecto de términos médicos (español-inglés).

Vocabulario bilingüe para la profesión médica está dividido en lecciones según el tema indicado. Los principales componentes de cada lección son: vocabularios, una o más conversaciones, apuntes gramaticales, una útil información adicional, un proyecto bilingüe (ejercicio preparatorio o transcripción) y ejercicios. Se recomienda que el estudiante se refiera al índice como guía de referencia.

Son los deseos del autor, querido estudiante, que al final del curso no sólo hayas aprendido la terminología y las expresiones relacionadas con el campo de la medicina, sino que también te haya ayudado en el aprendizaje de estos hermosos idiomas (español-inglés), y en la comprensión de las dos culturas a las cuales dan expresión.

R.E.

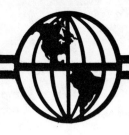

GREETINGS
SALUDOS Y DESPEDIDAS

VOCABULARY — VOCABULARIO

A. Medical—Médico

clínica	— clinic
dolor	— pain
enfermedad	— sickness, illness
enfermero, enfermera	— nurse
hospital	— hospital
medicina	— medicine
médico, doctor	— doctor, physician, M.D.
paciente	— patient

B. General

cama	— bed
¿cómo?	— How?
cuarto	— room
día	— day
el, la, los, las	— the
esposo	— husband
familia	— family
hay	— there is, there are
hijo (s)	— child, children
libro	— book
mesa	— table
noche	— night
pared	— wall
pizarra	— blackboard
reloj	— watch, clock
señor	— mister, Mr.
señora	— madam, Mrs.
señorita	— miss
tarde	— afternoon
tiza	— chalk
un, una, unos, unas	— a, an, some
ventana	— window

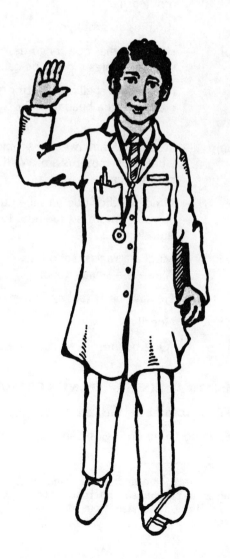

CONVERSATION — CONVERSACION*

A. Dr. Robert Lamp enters the room in the hospital to see a patient, Manuel Payán, and the nurse, Lucila Maury, does the necessary translating.

El Dr. Robert Lamp entra al cuarto en el hospital para ver a un paciente, Manuel Payán; y la enfermera, Lucila Maury, hace la traducción necesaria.

Dr. Lamp	— Good morning, Manuel, How are you today?	*Buenos días, Manuel, ¿cómo está usted hoy?*
Lucila	— Buenos días, Manuel, ¿cómo está usted hoy?	
Manuel	— Estoy un poco mejor, pero no del todo bien.	*I'm a little better, but not completely well.*
Lucila	— He says he feels a little better, but not completely well.	*Dice que se siente un poco mejor, pero no del todo bien.*
Dr. Lamp	— Please ask him what his problem is.	*Pregúntele, por favor, ¿cuál es su problema?*
Lucila	— ¿Cuál es su problema?	
Manuel	— Hace dos días que tengo desmayos, calambres y dolor de cabeza.	*For two days I've had spells of fainting, cramps, and a headache.*
Lucila	— He has had spells of fainting, cramps and a headache for two days.	*Ha tenido ...*
Dr. Lamp	— Please tell him we already know what his symptoms are. We'll take care of him.	*Dígale por favor, que ya sabemos cuáles son sus síntomas. Nosotros lo atenderemos.*
Lucila	— El doctor dice que ya sabe cuáles son sus síntomas, que aquí lo atenderemos.	
Manuel	— Muchas gracias, señorita. Ahora me siento mejor.	*Thank you, miss, I feel better now.*
Lucila	— He says he is feeling better now.	*Dice que ahora se siente mejor.*
Dr. Lamp	— Good!	*¡Qué bueno!*
Lucila	— ¡Qué bueno!	

GRAMMATICAL HINTS — APUNTES GRAMATICALES*

A. El verbo **to be** — the verb **to be.**

El verbo **to be** en inglés tiene una sola conjugación y no constituye mayor problema.

---

* The Conversations and other similar materials contained in each lesson alternate with the Grammatical Hints that also form part of the same lesson.

* Las conversaciones, así como cualesquier otro material que se incluye en esta parte de cada una de las lecciones, se alterna sucesivamente con los apuntes gramaticales de la misma.

B. In Spanish there are two verbs which mean **to be**. Each verb has definite uses which cannot be interchanged. In this lesson we will concentrate on the verb **estar** and the verb **ser** will appear in the following lesson. The verb **to be** is conjugated in the following manner.

I am	— yo soy - estoy
you are	— tú eres - estás
	— usted es - está
	— ustedes son - están
he, she, it, is	— él, ella es - está
we are	— nosotros, nosotras somos - estamos
they are	— ellos, ellas son - están

The most common uses of **estar** in Spanish are:

1. To indicate temporary state or condition.
e.g. ¿Cómo está usted hoy?   — How are you today?
Estoy bien gracias   — I'm well, thank you.

2. To indicate location whether temporary or permanent.
e.g. Los pacientes están en el hospital — The patients are in the hospital.

3. In the progressive form: e.g. Estoy leyendo — I am reading.

CONVERSATION — CONVERSACION (Cont.)

B. Miss Margarita Díaz happens to meet Mrs. Sonia Fisher, who is with a friend who just came from Texas; her name is Patricia Barr.

La señorita Margarita Díaz se encuentra con la señora Sonia Fisher que está con una amiga que acaba de llegar de Texas; su nombre es Patricia Barr.

Margarita — ¿Cómo está, señora Fisher? Hace (hacía) tiempo que no la veo (veía).

How are you Mrs. Fisher?
I haven't seen you for a long time.

Sonia — Buenas tardes, Margarita. Me da gusto verte. ¿qué tal?

Good afternoon, Margarita.
I am happy to see you, how are things going?

Margarita — Todo está bien, y ¿cómo están por su casa?

Everything is all right, and how is everybody at home?

Sonia — Todos estamos bien. Margarita, te presento a mi amiga Patricia que acaba de llegar de Texas.

We're all fine. Margarita, I would like to introduce my friend Patricia to you; she just came from Texas.

Margarita — Mucho gusto.

My pleasure.

Sonia — She says she is very happy to meet you.

Dice que está muy contenta de conocerla.

Patricia — I am very happy, too.

Y yo también.

Sonia — Ella está contenta también.

She is also happy.

Margarita — ¿Qué profesión tiene?

What's her profession?

Sonia — Es enfermera.

She is a nurse.

GRAMMATICAL HINTS — APUNTES GRAMATICALES (Cont.)

C. Definite Articles — Artículos definidos

All nouns in Spanish have gender and number. Each noun is either masculine or feminine, singular or plural (one or more than one).

1. If a noun ends in **o** it is normally considered masculine, and has the article **el** before it if it is singular and **los** if it is plural.

e.g. **el** libro — the book   **los** libros — **the** books.

2. If a noun ends in **e** or in a consonant, it may be either masculine or feminine.
It is important for the students to learn each noun together with its gender.

3. If a noun ends in **a** it is normally considered feminine and takes the article **la** if singular and **las** if plural.

e.g. **la** señorita — miss   **las** señoritas — misses (the young ladies).
   la enfermera — **the** nurse   **las** enfermeras — **the** nurses.

el				la		
	doctor	— doctor			doctora	— doctor
	esposo	— husband			esposa	— wife
	hijo	— son			hija	— daughter
	señor	— mister, gentleman			señora	— Mrs., lady
	libro	— book			casa	— house
	cuarto	— room			cama	— bed
	banco	— bank			familia	— family

D. Artículos definidos — Definite articles

1. El artículo definido **el, la, los, las (the)**, se usa más en español que en inglés.

2. Este artículo se usa tanto en masculino como en femenino, singular o plural.
   e.g. **The** desk — **El** escritorio   **The** universities — **Las** universidades.

CONVERSATION — CONVERSACION (Cont.)

C. The English professor asks his **Latino** students the following questions.

El profesor de inglés le hace **a** sus estudiantes **latinos** las siguientes preguntas:

Professor — Francisco, do you understand English?

Francisco, ¿entiende Ud. inglés?

Francisco — Un poquito, profesor.

Just a little.

Professor — In English.

En inglés.

Francisco — Just a little.

Professor — Inés, what does "please" mean?

Inés, ¿qué significa la palabra "please"?

Inés — Hable más despacio, por favor.

Please speak more slowly.

Professor — You already gave the meaning. Carlos, how do you say "doctor", "hospital", "paciente", "enfermera", and "cama" in English?

Ud. acaba de dar el significado. Carlos, ¿cómo se dice en inglés...?

Carlos	— Professor, you say "doctor" "hospital", "patient", "nurse", and "bed".	*En inglés se dice ...*
Professor	— Very well. Justo, how do you express gratitude?	*Justo, ¿cómo se dan las gracias?*
Justo	— By saying "thank you".	*Diciendo "thank you".*
Professor	— Celisa, what does "my deepest sympathy" mean?	*Celisa, ¿qué significa la expresión "my deepest sympathy"?*
Celisa	— Repita otra vez, por favor.	*Repeat, please.*
Professor	— "My deepest sympathy".	
Celisa	— I don't know.	*Yo no sé.*
Professor	— Tell her, Juan.	*Dígale, Juan.*
Juan	— Mi más sentido pésame.	
Celisa	— Gracias.	*Thank you.*
Professor	— Luis, did you bring your assignment?	*Luis, trajo usted su tarea?*
Luis	— I am sorry, but I didn't bring it.	*Lo siento mucho, pero no la traje.*
Professor	— That is a bad excuse, but good English. All of you bring your assignment tomorrow.	*Esa es una mala excusa, aunque dicha en buen inglés. Traigan todos la tarea para mañana.*

GRAMMATICAL HINTS — APUNTES GRAMATICALES (Cont.)

E. Artículos indefinidos — Indefinite articles

1. Los artículos indefinidos se usan más en inglés que en español.
Estos artículos son: **a, an,** (un, una, unos, unas).

2. El artículo **a** se usa ante el sonido de una consonante.
e.g. a book — un libro.
An se usa ante el sonido de una vocal.
e.g. an apple — una manzana.

F. Indefinite articles — Artículos indefinidos

1. The article **un** precedes a masculine singular noun and **unos** a masculine plural noun.
e.g. un médico — a doctor.
unos remedios — some (a few) medicines.

2. The article **una** precedes a feminine singular noun and **unas** a feminine plural noun.
e.g. una mesa — a table.
unas enfermeras — some (a few) nurses.

G. Contractions — Contracciones

1. There are only two contractions in Spanish: **al** and **del.**
a + el = **al,** e.g. voy al pueblo — I am going to town.
de + el = **del,** e.g. vengo del pueblo — I come from town.

2. En inglés hay muchas contracciones las cuales serán explicadas más adelante.

H. Subject pronouns — Pronombres personales

1. The subject pronouns in Spanish are:*

yo — I
tú — you (this is a familiar form used in the singular), **fam.** (=familiar), **sing.** (=singular).
él — he
ella — she
usted — you (this is a formal form used in the singular), **for.** (=formal)
nosotros, nosotras — we
ustedes — (this from is used in the plural). **plu.** (= plural)
ellos, ellas — they

2. Tú se usa en la forma familiar mientras que usted (Ud.) se usa en la forma formal. En inglés no hay problema alguno porque hay sólo una forma.

ADDITIONAL INFORMATION — INFORMACION ADICIONAL

1. Useful expressions — Expresiones útiles

adiós	— good by	hasta luego	— so long
buena suerte	— good luck	hasta mañana	— see you tomorrow
buenas noches	— good evening, good	hasta pronto	— see you later
	night	hola	— hi, hello
buenas tardes	— good afternoon	muy bien	— very good
buenos días	— good morning	nos vemos	— we'll see you
con mucho gusto	— my pleasure	perdóneme	— excuse me
el placer es mío	— the pleasure is mine	por favor	— please

2. Idiomatic expressions — Expresiones idiomáticas

a la orden, de nada	— you're welcome	gozar de	— to enjoy
		gracias	— thank you
darse cuenta	— to realize	tener éxito	— to be successful
enamorarse de	— to fall in love with	tener una cita	— to have an engagement or
en efecto	— in fact, in effect		appointment
faltar a una cita	— to break an engagement		

3. Numbers — Números

1. uno	— one		11. once	— eleven
2. dos	— two		12. doce	— twelve
3. tres	— three		13. trece	— thirteen
4. cuatro	— four		14. catorce	— fourteen
5. cinco	— five		15. quince	— fifteen
6. seis	— six		16. dieciséis	— sixteen
7. siete	— seven		17. diecisiete	— seventeen
8. ocho	— eight		18. dieciocho	— eighteen
9. nueve	— nine		19. diecinueve	— nineteen
10. diez	— ten		20. veinte	— twenty

---

* There is another subject pronoun: **Vosotros** (you **fam. plu.**).
That is used only in Spain. Therefore we are not going to use it in this book.

$5 + 4 = 9$ cinco y cuatro son 9 — five and four are nine
$6 + 2 = 8$ seis más dos son ocho — six plus two are eight
$10 - 3 = 7$ diez menos tres son siete — ten minus (less) three are seven.

4. Spanish names — Nombres hispanos

Alberto	Inés
Antonio	Loyda
Celisa	Mario
Cristina	Pablo
Dolores, Lola	Pedro
Elena	Rafael
Gloria	Ricardo
Guadalupe (Lupe)	Rosa

Nombres ingleses —English names

Albert	Ben
Alice	Betty
Andrew	Beverly
Ann	Bill
Arthur	Bonnie
Barbara	Brad
Barry	Colleen
Becky	Heather

5. Questions — Preguntas

¿Cómo le va? — How is it going?
¿Cómo marcha todo? — How is everything?
¿Cómo se siente? — How do you feel?
¿Qué es esto?   — What is this?

Es el abdomen	— It is the abdomen	Es la boca	— It is the mouth
el brazo	— the arm	la cabeza	— the head
el cuello	— the neck	la columna	
el estómago	— the stomach	vertebral	— the spinal column
el hombro	— the shoulder	la espalda	— the back
el labio	— the lip	la lengua	— the tongue
el ojo	— the eye	la mano	— the hand
el pecho	— the chest	la mejilla	— the cheek
el pie	— the foot	la nariz	— the nose
el tobillo	— the ankle	la nuca	— the nape of the neck
		la rodilla	— the knee

BILINGUAL PROJECT — PROYECTO BILINGUE

PREPARATORY EXERCISE 1 — EJERCICIO PREPARATORIO 1

(Students learning Spanish and students learning English).

The first exercise of each of the first 10 lessons of this text is called a **Preparatory Exercise.** Each **Preparatory Exercise** consists of a resume, report, or form to be filled out which is of the type usually required of medical-secretarial personnel.

The **Preparatory Exercise** of the first three lessons are completed for you: these are models; you, the student, are not to repeat the same information. Your job in each case is to write out your own report, to design and fill out your own forms, etc., on the basis of your own or someone else's experience as a sick perso

(Estudiantes de español y estudiantes de inglés).

El primer ejercicio de cada una de las diez primeras lecciones de este texto se llama **ejercicio preparatorio.** Según sea el caso, cada **ejercicio preparatorio** consiste o, en un resumen, un informe, o un formulario a llenar, los cuales por regla general corresponden a los que toda secretaria (o) u oficinista médico tiene que preparar en su práctica profesional.

Los **ejercicios preparatorios** de las tres primeras lecciones se presentan en su forma final: son modelos; usted, el estudiante, no debería de repetir la misma información. El cometido suyo, en cada caso, consiste en redactar su propio

Family members and friends can be of great help here. You may of course draw heavily upon your own general medical knowledge and your own imagination as you try to envision each situation and how to describe it within the framework of the model reports and forms that the text provides you as a pattern and reference.

It is recommended that each student do these exercises in both languages, if such is feasible.

As regards this initial **Preparatory Exercise,** write out a simple report of a case history using the format and the headings that appear below.

informe, preparar su propio modelo de formulario, para después llenarlo, etc., valiéndose de su propia experiencia o de la de otra persona, familiar o amigo. Evidentemente, le corresponde a cada estudiante echar mano de sus conocimientos médicos en general y usar de su propia imaginación al tratar de visualizar cada situación, y determinar cómo ésta debe ser descrita dentro del marco de los informes y formularios modelo que ofrece el texto como patrones y referencias. Se recomienda que cada alumno trate de hacer estos ejercicios en ambos idiomas, si le es posible.

En cuanto a este ejercicio preparatorio inicial, escriba un informe sencillo de una historia clínica, empleando el formato y los títulos que aparecen a continuación.

NAME — NOMBRE _____

ADDRESS — DIRECCION _____

_____

DATE — FECHA _____

PHYSICIAN — DOCTOR(A) _____

HOSPITAL — HOSPITAL _____

DATE OF BIRTH — FECHA DE NACIMIENTO _____

OCCUPATION — OCUPACION _____

RACE — RAZA _____

CHIEF COMPLAINT — SINTOMA PRINCIPAL _____

_____

HISTORY OF PRESENT ILLNESS — HISTORIA DE LA ENFERMEDAD ACTUAL _____

_____

FAMILY HISTORY — HISTORIA DE LA FAMILIA _____

_____

PHYSICAL DIAGNOSIS — DIAGNOSTICO FISICO _____

TREATMENT PRESCRIBED — TRATAMIENTO INDICADO _____

_____

EXERCISES — EJERCICIOS

(Students learning Spanish — Estudiantes de español)

A. Translate into Spanish.

1. The patient is sick. ....

2. I am very well, thank you. ....

3. How do you say this?. ....

4. What is this?. ....

5. Ten plus 25 is 35. ....

6. She is there. ....

7. He is all right. ....

8. This is a book. ....

9. Where is your head?. ....

10. You are feeling well. ....

B. Fill in the blanks with the correct article, if necessary.

1. Yo tengo _____ buen radio.

2. Hoy es _____ miércoles.

3. No tenemos clases _____ domingos.

4. Me gustan _____ deportes.

5. _____ Dr. Smith está aquí.

6. Ella es _____ mexicana.

7. Son _____ nueve.

8. Hay _____ libro en la mesa.

9. Ella viene de _____ Argentina.

10. El es _____ buen chico.

11. Me duele _____ cabeza.

12. El tiene una inflamación en _____ nariz.

13. _____ corazón es un órgano muy importante.

14. Nosotros estudiamos _____ español.

C. Write six complete sentences in Spanish with the idiomatic expressions given in the additional information.

1. ....   4. ....

2. ....   5. ....

3. ....   6. ....

D. Answer the following questions in complete Spanish.

1. Buenos días, ¿cómo está usted hoy? ....

2. ¿Cómo se siente el paciente? ....

3. ¿Dónde está el hospital? ....

4. ¿Cuántos son seis más once? ....

5. ¿Qué es esto? ....

EJERCICIOS — EXERCISES

(Estudiantes de inglés — Students learning English)

A. Traduzca al inglés.

1. Con mucho gusto. ....

2. Buenos días, ¿cómo está el paciente? ....

3. ¿Dónde está el doctor? ....

4. La señora está enferma. ....

5. Te veo. ....

6. Buena suerte. ....

7. 20 menos 12 son ocho. ....

8. Hasta mañana ....

9. ¿Dónde está su nariz? ....

10. Esto es un libro. ....

B. Llene los espacios vacíos con el artículo correspondiente, si es necesario.

1. I like _____ sports.

2. We are going to see _____ Dr. Díaz.

3. She doesn't work on _____ Sundays.

4. The nurse is _____ Catholic.

5. He is _____ Mexican.

6. It's _____ 9:30.

7. The doctor is _____ good man.

8. I have _____ headache.

9. Today is _____ Tuesday.

10. I have _____ car.

11. _____ head is a part of the body.

12. We are studying _____ English.

13. There is _____ watch on the wall.

14. They don't like _____ medicine.

C. Escriba seis oraciones completas en inglés con algunas expresiones idiomáticas dadas en la información adicional.

1. ....   4. ....

2. ....   5. ....

3. ....   6. ....

D. Conteste a las siguientes preguntas en inglés.

1. How do you feel today? ....

2. Where is your book? ....

3. How is everything at home? ....

4. What's that? ....

5. How is the professor? ....

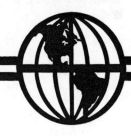

HOME AND FAMILY
EL HOGAR Y LA FAMILIA

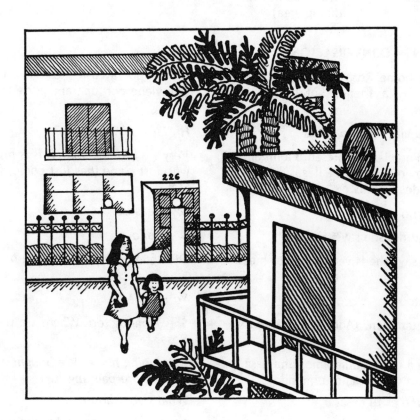

VOCABULARY — VOCABULARIO

A. Medical — Médico

aguja	— needle	antibiótico	— antibiotic
alergia	— allergy	diabetes	— diabetes
alérgico	— allergic	enfermo (a)	— a patient, sick
algodón	— cotton	epiléptico	— epileptic
amígdalas	— tonsils	supervisor (a)	— supervisor

B. General

alcoba, dormitorio	— bedroom	cuarto	— room
ascendencia	— ancestry	despensa	— storeroom, pantry
azul	— blue	difícil	— difficult
baño	— bath, bathroom	fácil	— easy
blanco (a)	— white	grande	— big
bonito (a)	— pretty, cute	hermoso (a)	— beautiful, hand-some, good-look-ing
cocina	— kitchen		
cómodo (a)	— comfortable		
¿Cuántos?	— How many?	mayor	— older, larger

menor	— younger, smaller	simpático (a)	— nice, pleasant, congenial, engaging, amusing
muy	— very		
negro (a)	— black	también	— also
pequeño (a)	— little, small		
rojo (a)	— red		
sala-comedor	— living room (with dining area)		

CONVERSATION — CONVERSACION

A. On her way home Rosa meets Lilia, who is acompanied by a friend, Kathy, from the United States.

Volviendo a casa, Rosa se encuentra con Lilia, que viene con una amiga de los Estados Unidos.

Rosa — Hola Lilia, ¿cómo estás?

Hi, Lilia, how are you?

Lilia — Bien gracias. Te presento a mi amiga Kathy que acaba de llegar de los Estados Unidos.

Very well, thank you. This is my friend, Kathy, who just came (has just come) from the United States.

Rosa — Mucho gusto.

My pleasure.

Kathy — What did she say?

¿Qué dijo?

Lilia — She says she is very happy to meet you.

Dice que está muy contenta de conocerte.

Kathy — Me too.

Yo también.

Lilia — Ella también. ¿Adónde vas ahora?

She is happy too. Where are you going now, Rosa?

Rosa — Voy a casa. Compramos una casa nueva y la estamos pintando.

I am going home. We bought a new house and we are painting it.

Lilia — ¿Cómo es tu casa?

What's your house like?

Rosa — Mi casa es grande y bonita. Tiene tres dormitorios, una cocina, una sala, dos baños y un garaje doble. ¿Cómo es la tuya y la de Kathy?

My house is large and beautiful. It has three bedrooms, a kitchen, a living room, two baths, and a double garage. What is yours and Kathy's like?

Lilia — La mía es pequeña. Kathy, what is your house like?

Mine is small. Kathy, ¿cómo es tu casa?

Kathy — We don't have a house in the States, we have a condominium.

No tenemos una casa en los Estados Unidos, tenemos un condominio.

Lilia — No tienen una casa sino un condominio.

They don't have a house but rather a condominium.

Rosa — Muy interesante. Ahora tengo que irme. Adiós.

Very interesting, I have to go. Good-by.

Lilia — Adiós.

Kathy — By.

GRAMMATICAL HINTS — APUNTES GRAMATICALES

A. We have already mentioned in Lesson One that the English verb **to be** has two possibilities in Spanish; **ser** and **estar.** You are already familiar with **estar** and its uses. The uses of the verb **ser** are the following:

1. To indicate inherent or relatively permanent qualities of the subject.
   e.g. Mi casa es grande — My house is big.

2. With the preposition **de** to indicate:
   a) Origin
      e.g. Tú eres de España — You are from Spain.
   b) Possesion
      e.g. El libro es del doctor — The book is the doctor's.
   c) Material from which an object is made
      e.g. La casa es de madera — The house is (made) of wood.

3. To indicate the hour of the day.
   e.g. ¿Qué hora es? — What time is it?

B. Oraciones afirmativas

Las oraciones afirmativas se forman en inglés tal como en español, con la diferencia de que en inglés, cuando se quiere dar énfasis a la frase, se pone el auxiliar **do o does** (tercera persona singular) en el presente y **did** en el pasado. Este auxiliar va antes del verbo.
e.g. I **do** like it — Me gusta mucho (en verdad).
   He **does** work — El trabaja (de veras).

C. Oraciones negativas

1. Para transformar una oración afirmativa en negativa se coloca la palabra **not** después del verbo **to be.** También se usan las contracciones **isn't** o **aren't.**
   e.g. He is not an executive — El no es un ejecutivo.

2. Con otros verbos se colocan las siguientes palabras: **do not** o **does not,** o las contracciones **don't** o **doesn't** antes del verbo.
   e.g. I don't like it — No me gusta.
      He didn't go — El no fue.

3. Con el verbo **to have** y otros verbos auxiliares como **can,** se puede poner la terminación negativa al final o su contracción negativa.
   e.g. I haven't done it — No lo he hecho.
   Con el verbo **can** (poder — nótese que no se dice "to can"). En el caso de **can,** también se dice **cannot.**
   e.g. I can't do it — No puedo hacerlo.

CONVERSATION — CONVERSACION (Cont.)

B. Peter and Luke are social workers; and Peter, who had a minor in Spanish while in college, does all the translating while they visit Gonzalo Contreras.

Peter y Luke son trabajadores sociales, y Peter, que estudió español mientras asistía a la universidad, traduce todo mientras visitan a Gonzalo Contreras.

Peter — Buenos días, señor Contreras, ¿cómo está usted hoy?

Good morning, Mr. Contreras, how are you today?

Gonzalo — Regular.

Just fair.

Luke	— Tell him we are social workers, and we would like to ask him some questions.	*Dile que nosotros somos trabajadores sociales y que quisiéramos hacerle algunas preguntas.*
Peter	— Nosotros somos trabajadores sociales y quisiéramos hacerle algunas preguntas.	
Gonzalo	— Está bien.	*Very well.*
Peter	— He is ready.	*El está dispuesto a contestar.*
Luke	— Mr. Contreras, how many members are there in your family?	
Peter	— Sr. Contreras, ¿cuántas personas hay en su familia?	
Gonzalo	— Somos ocho por todos.	*There are eight of us in all.*
Luke	— Who are they?	
Peter	— ¿Quiénes son?	
Gonzalo	— Mi esposa, yo, y nuestros seis hijos.	*My wife, myself, and our six children.*
Peter	— His wife, himself, and their six children.	*Su esposa, él y sus seis hijos.*
Luke	— How many members of the family are working?	
Peter	— ¿Cuántos miembros de su familia trabajan?	
Gonzalo	— Solamente yo.	*I am the only one.*
Peter	— He is the only one.	*El es el único.*
Luke	— All right. We have all the information. Thank you.	*Muy bien. Hemos obtenido toda la información. Gracias.*
Peter	— Muchas gracias por su colaboración.	*Thank you for your cooperation.*
Gonzalo	— A sus órdenes.	*You are welcome.*

APPOINTMENT — CITA

> Dr. Frank Beiley
> 100 Canyon Rd.
> Napa, CA 94558
> Telephone (707) 252-7705
>
> For_____
> Para_____
>
> Date_____ at:_____ o'clock
>
> Fecha_____ a las_____
>
> If unable to keep appointment, kindly give 24 hours notice.
> Si no puede cumplir con la cita, favor de avisarnos con 24 horas de anticipación.

CONVERSATION — CONVERSACION (Cont.)

C. In the hospital the supervisor asks the nurse:

En el hospital la supervisora le pregunta a la enfermera:

Supervisora — Who are the patients in room 15?	¿Quiénes son los pacientes del cuarto número 15?
Enfermera — They are Puerto Rican patients.	Son pacientes puertorriqueños.
Supervisora — Do they know English?	¿Saben inglés?
Enfermera — No.	
Supervisora — Vamos allá.	Let's go there.
(They go to the room.)	(Van al cuarto).
Enfermera — Buenas tardes, señores, ¿cómo están ustedes?	Good afternoon, gentlemen, how are you?
Francisco — Pues, señorita, yo estoy un poco mejor, pero mi compañero está grave.	I feel better, but my roommate is in serious condition.
Enfermera — He says he is doing all right, but his roommate is in serious condition.	
Supervisora — Then we must place them in different rooms.	Entonces hay que ponerlos en cuartos diferentes.
Francisco — ¿Qué dice ella?	What is she saying?
Enfermera — Dice que los van a poner en cuartos diferentes.	
Francisco — Buena idea.	Good idea.

ADDITIONAL INFORMATION — INFORMACION ADICIONAL

1. Useful expressions — Expresiones útiles

¿Cómo se llama usted? — What's your name?
¿Es usted casado? — Are you married?
¿En qué puedo servirle? — May I help you?
Llene esto, por favor — Please fill this out.
¿Cuál es su domicilio (dirección)? — What's your address?
¿Cuál es su número de teléfono? — What's your phone number?
¿Cuántos años tiene? — How old are you?
¿Cuál es el apellido de su madre? — What's your mother's last name?
¿Quién es su pariente más cercano? — Who's your closest relative?
¿Es usted alérgico a alguna cosa? — Are you allergic to anything?

2. Idiomatic expressions — Expresiones idiomáticas

acabar de	— to have just	entonces	— then
a propósito	— by the way	la semana entrante	— next week
ayer	— yesterday	mañana	— tomorrow
dolor de cabeza	— headache	tener que	— to have to

3. Spanish Names — Nombres hispanos

Antonia	Jaime
Armando	José
Daniel	Luis
Esperanza	Margarita
Gloria	Roberto
Isaías	Rogelio

Nombres ingleses — English names

Brenda	Carol
Brian	Carolyn
Bruce	Catherine
Caren	Charlene
Carl	Charles
Carla	Craig

4. Relatives — Familiares (parientes)

abuela	— grandmother		nuera	— daughter-in-law
abuelos	— grandparents		padrastro	— stepfather
cuñada	— sister-in-law		padres	— parents
cuñado	— brother-in-law		padrino	— godfather
esposa	— wife		prima	— cousin (female)
esposo	— husband		primo	— cousin (male)
familiares	— family members		sobrina	— niece
hija	— daughter		sobrino	— nephew
hijo	— son		suegra	— mother-in-law
madrastra	— stepmother		suegro	— father-in-law
madrina	— godmother		tía	— aunt
novia	— girlfriend		tío	— uncle
novio	— boyfriend		yerno	— son-in-law

5. Numbers — Números

21 veintiuno	— twenty-one		26 veintiséis	— twenty-six
22 veintidós	— twenty-two		27 veintisiete	— twenty-seven
23 veintitrés	— twenty-three		28 veintiocho	— twenty-eight
24 veinticuatro	— twenty-four		29 veintinueve	— twenty-nine
25 veinticinco	— twenty-five		30 treinta	— thirty

6. More parts of a house — Más partes de la casa

azotea	— flat roof		jardín	— garden
biblioteca	— library		oficina	— office
comedor	— dining room		patio	— patio
dos pisos	— two stories		pórtico	— porch
escalera	— stairs		recámara	— bedroom
garage	— garage		sótano	— basement

BILINGUAL PROJECT — PROYECTO BILINGUE

PREPARATORY EXERCISE 2 — EJERCICIO PREPARATORIO 2

APPOINTMENT BOOK — LIBRETA DE CITAS

Appointments are made with a pencil instead of a pen. The secretary should plan the appointments so that unused time can be filled easily.

Each patient requires a 30-minute appointment. (See example on next page).

Las citas se escriben con lápiz en vez de pluma. La secretaria debe hacer las citas de tal forma que el tiempo libre se pueda aprovechar fácilmente.

Cada paciente requiere una cita de unos 30 minutos. (Vea ejemplo en pág 17).

EXAMPLE (Appointment Book) — **EJEMPLO** (Libro de citas).

TUESDAY   MARTES

Time		3/5				3/5	
8:00							
15							
30							
45							
9:00		ROUNDS				RONDAS	
15							
30							
45							
10:00	Mrs. Jayne Thorp	Treatment - head	965-2373		Sra. Jayne Thorp	Tratamiento - cabeza	965-2373
15	Miss Joy Lee	chg dressing +	433-4321		Srta. Joy Lee	Cambio de vendajes	433-4321
30		examination and				examen y	
45		counseling				consejo	
11:00	Mr. Thomas Don	P.E.	725-3241		Sr. Thomas Don	Examen físico	725-3241
15							
30							
45	Mrs. Lena Moore	P.E. and Pap S.	932-4521		Sra. Lena Moore	Examen físico y	932-4521
12:00						papanicolao	
15							
30	Luncheon meet				Reunión y		
45	Hilton Hotel				almerzo en el		
1:00					Hotel Hilton		
15							
30							
45							
2:00	Mr. Pierre-Louis	Skin ex.	565-2435		Sr. Pierre-Louis	Examen de la piel	565-2435
15							
30	Mr. John Fisher	EKG and interpretation	240-5655		Sr. John Fisher	ECG e interpretación	240-5655
45							
3:00	Mrs. Jeanine Smith	IUD INSERTION	942-5870		Sra. Jeanine Smith	Inserción de IUD	942-5870
15							
30	Miss Nancy Long	PE and Pap S.	433-6540		Srta. Nancy Long	Examen físico y	433-6540
45						papanicolao	
4:00							
15	Mr. Joel Brown	Treatment - head	491-6159		Sr. Joel Brown	Tratamiento - cabeza	491-6159
30	Mrs. Janice Carter	chg dressing	914-4513		Sra. Janice Carter	Cambio de vendajes	914-4513
45							
5:00	OPEN TIME				TIEMPO LIBRE		
15							
30							
45							

Make your own program for Wednesday — Haga su propio programa para el miércoles.

EXERCISES — EJERCICIOS

(Students learning Spanish — Estudiantes de español)

A. Fill in the blanks with the correct form of ser.

1. El _____ médico.

2. Pablo y María _____ salvadoreños.

3. Yo _____ estudiante.

4. Tú _____ enfermera.

5. Lupe y yo _____ profesores.

6. El doctor _____ simpático

7. Esta lección _____ también fácil.

8. Los libros _____ azules.

9. ¿Cómo _____ tu casa?

10. Hoy _____ martes.

B. Translate the following sentences.

1. She is a Mexican. ....

2. We are North Americans. ....

3. The patient is allergic to antibiotics. ....

4. My grandfather is epileptic. ....

5. She is of Spanish ancestry. ....

C. Answer the following questions in complete Spanish.

1. ¿Cómo está Ud. hoy? ....

2. ¿Cuántos miembros hay en su familia? ....

3. ¿Cómo es su hermana? ....

4. ¿Cuántos hermanos mayores hay en su familia? ....

D. Write six sentences with some of the idiomatic expressions.

1. ....

2. ....

3. ....

4. ....

5. ....

6. ....

EJERCICIOS — EXERCISES

(Estudiantes de inglés — Students learning English)

A. Cambie las oraciones siguientes a su forma negativa.

1. We like fruits. ....

2. Today is Friday. ....

3. You are a student. ....

4. The secretary works hard. ....

5. The boss is in his office. ....

B. Cambie las siguientes palabras a la forma plural.

1. Office ....

2. Secretary ....

3. Housewife ....

4. Foreman ....

5. Dolly ....

6. Boss ....

7. Laboratory ....

8. Life ....

9. Client ....

10. Capital ....

11. Manuscript ....

12. Church ....

C. Traduzca las siguientes oraciones.

1. Los pacientes son mexicanos. ....
2. Buena idea. ....
3. Hay cuatro miembros en mi familia. ....
4. Yo no soy un trabajador social. ....
5. Mi casa es pequeña y bonita. ....
6. Estoy muy contento de conocerle. ....
7. Mi casa tiene cuatro dormitorios. ....
8. ¿Sabe usted inglés? ....
9. ¿Cómo están sus padres? ....
10. ¿El enfermo está en el hospital ....

D. Conteste en inglés

1. Where is your house? ....
2. How is your family? ....
3. What is your house like? ....
4. How many members are there in your family? ....
5. Who is your sister? ....

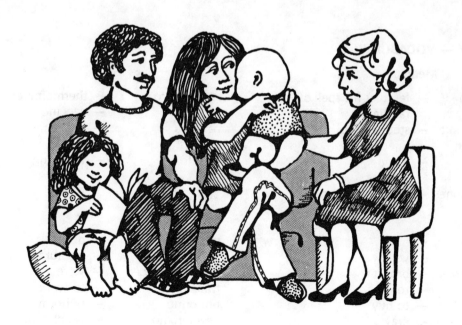

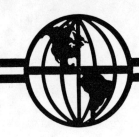

EVERYDAY ACTIVITIES
ACTIVIDADES DIARIAS

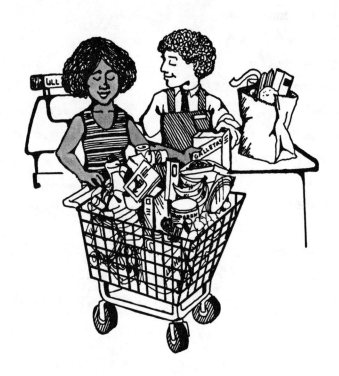

VOCABULARY — VOCABULARIO

A. Medical — Médico

desmayo	— fainting fit, spell of fainting	termómetro	— thermometer
estetoscopio	— stethoscope	vacuna	— vaccine
inyección	— injection	vértebra	— vertebra
nervio	— nerve	virus	— virus
sala de operaciones	— operating room	vómito	— vomiting

B. General

ahora	— now	plato	— dish
amarillo	— yellow	restaurante	— restaurant
café, marrón	— brown	tienda, almacén	— store
comer	— to eat	trabajar	— to work
comprar	— to buy	uniforme	— uniform
gris	— gray	vegetariano	— vegetarian
necesitar	— to need	verde	— green
nuevo (a)	— new	vestido	— dress
partido	— game	viejo	— old

CONVERSATION — CONVERSACION

A. Julio meets Efrain and Lucy, a girl who is learning Spanish in the same university they all attend.

Julio   — Buenos días, ¿adónde van ustedes?

Efraín — Buenos días, Julio. Vamos a la universidad.

Lucy   — Good morning.

Julio   — Buenos días, señorita, ¿cómo anda su español?

Efraín — How is your Spanish going?

Lucy   — Muy … despacio.

Julio   — Muy bien, así es como se aprende.

Efraín — ¿Y tú adónde vas?

Julio   — Voy a un ensayo. Yo toco en la banda.

Efraín — ¿Qué piensas hacer esta noche?

Julio   — Nada en particular.

Efraín — ¿Estudiamos juntos?

Julio   — Con gusto. Te espero esta noche en mi casa. Trae a tu amiga.

Efraín — Lucy, would you like to study at his home tonight?

Lucy   — Con …mucho …gusto.

Julio   — Entonces los espero a las ocho.

Efraín — Allí estaremos.

Lucy   — Adiós …

Julio se encuentra con Efraín y Lucy, una muchacha que está aprendiendo español en la misma universidad a la que todos ellos asisten.

Good morning, where are you going?

Good morning, Julio. We are going to the university.

Good morning, miss, how is your Spanish going?

Very …slow

Good, that's the way to learn.

And where are you going?

I am going to a rehearsal. I play in the band.

What are you planning to do tonight?

Nothing in particular.

Shall we study together?

With pleasure. I'll be waiting for you at my house tonight. Bring your friend.

Lucy ¿te gustaría estudiar en su casa esta noche?

Then I'll be waiting for you at eight.

We'll be there.

GRAMMATICAL HINTS — APUNTES GRAMATICALES

A. The conjugation of the verb **ir** goes like this:

yo voy	I go	I am going
tú vas	you (fam.) go	you (fam.) are going
usted va	you (for.) go	you (for.) are going
él, ella va	he, she goes	he, she is going
nosotros (as) vamos	we go	we are going
ellos, ellas van	they go	they are going
ustedes van	you (plural)	you are going

The verb **ir** requires the preposition **a** after it.
When the following noun is masculine singular the **a** combines with **el** to form **al.**

e.g. voy **a** la biblioteca — I am going to the library.
Ricardo va **al** pueblo — Ricardo is going to town.

B. El verbo **to go** se usa principalmente en inglés en la forma progresiva.
e.g. He is going to his house — Va a su casa.

to es el equivalente de la preposición **a** en español.

La preposición **a** se usa en español tal como **to** en inglés antes de un infinitivo.
e.g. I am going **to** study tonight — voy **a** estudiar esta noche.
Este verbo, tal como en español, se usa a menudo para expresar una idea en el futuro inmediato.
e.g. We are going to watch the movie tomorrow — Vamos a ver la película mañana.

CONVERSATION — CONVERSACION (Cont.)

B. Gloria meets Petra and John.

Gloria se encuentra con Petra y John.

| Gloria | — ¿De dónde vienen y adónde van tan a la carrera? | *Where are you coming from, and where are you going in such a hurry?* |

Petra — Venimos del trabajo y vamos a la tienda.

We are coming from work and we are going to the store.

Gloria — How are you John?

¿Cómo estás, Juan?

John — Very well, thank you.
I should say... "Bueno, gracias".

Bien, gracias.
¿Debiera decir ...?

Gloria — "Bien, gracias"

John — Bien, gracias... ¿Y... usted?

... And... you?

Petra — John está aprendiendo bastante español. Desde que comenzó a trabajar en el hospital lo practica bastante.

John is learning a lot of Spanish. Ever since he started working at the hospital he has been practicing a great deal.

John — Sí ... señorita.

Yes ... miss.

Gloria — ¿Qué van a hacer en la tienda?

What are you going to do at the store?

Petra — Vamos a comprar uniformes.
Los dos somos enfermeros.

We are going to buy uniforms. We both are nurses.

John — Enfermeros... no... enfermos.

(We are) nurses, not patients.

Gloria — ¡Qué chistoso!

How funny!

Petra — ¿Quieres venir con nosotros?

Do you want to come along?

Gloria — Con mucho gusto. Quiero comprar un vestido azul y unos zapatos negros.

With pleasure. I want to buy a blue dress and a pair of black shoes.

John — Yo necesitar ...zapatos... blancos

I need white shoes.

Petra — "Yo necesito", John...

John — "Yo necesito".

Petra	— Vamos.	*Let's go.*
John	— Vamos.	

GRAMMATICAL HINTS — APUNTES GRAMATICALES (Cont.)

C. The verb **tener** (to have) is conjugated in the following way.

yo tengo	— I have
tú tienes	— you (fam. sing.) have
usted tiene	— you (for. sing.) have
él, ella tiene	— he, she has
nosotros (as) tenemos	— we have
ellos, ellas tienen	— they have
ustedes tienen	— you **(fam. plur.)** have.

D. El verbo **to have** es más usado en español que en inglés, aunque se usa mucho también. **Tener que** se traduce **to have to.**

e.g. Tengo que ir a la tienda — I have to go to the store.

CONVERSATION — CONVERSACION (Cont.)

A. Fernando enters a restaurant with his girlfriend Gladys, who is learning Spanish.

Fernando entra a un restaurante acompañado de su novia Gladys, quien está estudiando español.

Fernando — Mozo, ¿tiene una mesa desocupada?

Waiter, do you have an empty table?

Mozo — Tengo varias. Allí hay una cerca de la ventana. ¿Se quieren sentar allí?

I have several. There is one by the window. Would you like to sit there?

Fernando — Gladys, would you like to sit by the window?

Gladys, ¿te quieres sentar cerca de la ventana?

Gladys — I would love to.

Me gustaría mucho.

(Se sientan, y luego viene el mozo a recibir la orden).

(They sit down, and then the waiter comes to take their order.)

Mozo — ¿En qué puedo servirles?

May I help you?

Fernando — La señorita quisiera un plato vegetariano y a mí me trae una paella, por favor.

The young lady would like to have a vegetarian plate, and I would like to have a "paella" (typical Spanish dish).

Mozo — ¿Qué van a tomar?

What are you going to drink?

Fernando — Gladys, what would you like to drink?

Gladys, ¿qué te gustaría tomar?

Gladys — A cold lemonade.

Una limonada fría.

Fernando — Tráiganos dos limonadas, por favor.

Please bring us two lemonades.

Mozo — ¿Es todo?

Is that all?

Fernando — Por lo pronto.

For the time being.

Mozo — Muy bien.

GRAMMATICAL HINTS — APUNTES GRAMATICALES (Cont.)

E. Preposiciones de lugar que se traducen como en.

1. La preposición **on** indica algo que toca una superficie.
e.g. The picture is **on** the wall.

2. In indica que algo está dentro de ciertos límites.
e.g. The flowers are **in** the vase.

3. At se usa con el nombre de un lugar específico o un punto local.
e.g. They are **at** home.

4. Otras preposiciones son:

from — de (procedencia)	— He is **from** Mexico.
of — de	— The table is **of** wood.
with — con	— He is going **with** Mary.
about — acerca de	— She asks **about** you.
to — a	— We are going **to** Argentina.

ADDITIONAL INFORMATION — INFORMACION ADICIONAL

1. Food — Comida

agua	— water	jugo	— juice
azúcar	— sugar	leche malteada	— milk shake
café	— coffee	legumbres, vegetales	— vegetables
caramelo	— candy	limonada	— lemonade
carne de pollo	— chicken	mantequilla	— butter
carne de res,		mantequilla de maní	— peanut butter
de vaca,	— beef	margarina	— margarine
chocolate	— chocolate or candy bar	mayonesa	— mayonnaise
dulce	— sweet	mermelada	— marmalade
flan	— custard	pan	— bread
fruta	— fruit	pudin, budín	— pudding
galleta	— cookie, cracker	sal	— salt
helado	— ice cream	soda, gaseosa	— soda pop
huevos	— eggs	sopa	— soup
jalea	— jelly	tallarines, espaguetis	— spaghetti

2. More vocabulary — Más vocabulario

aceite de cocinar	— cooking oil	calabaza	— squash, pumpkin
aceite de oliva	— olive oil	cebollas	— onions
aguacate	— avocado	cena	— supper
albaricoques,		cerezas	— cherries
chabacanos	— apricots	ciruelas	— plums
alcachofa	— artichoke	coliflor	— cauliflower
almuerzo	— lunch	crema	— cream
apio	— celery	cuchara	— spoon
arroz	— rice	cuchillo	— knife
bananas	— bananas	dátiles	— dates
bizcocho	— biscuit	desayuno	— breakfast

economía doméstica	— home economics	peras	— pears
espárragos	— asparagus	plátanos	— plantains
fresas	— strawberries	plato	— plate
galletas de soda	— soda crackers	pollo	— chicken
gelatina	— gelatin	postre	— dessert
guisantes	— peas	propina	— tip
habichuelas	— string beans	queso	— cheese
harina	— flour	rábanos	— radishes
higos	— figs	remolacha	— beets
ingredientes	— ingredients	repollo	— cabbage
lechuga	— lettuce	requesón	— cottage cheese
lentejas	— lentils	sandía	— watermelon
limón	— lemon	sardinas	— sardines
maíz	— corn	servilleta	— napkin
manzanas	— apples	soya	— soybeans
melón	— cantaloupe	tenedor	— fork
menú	— menu	tomate	— tomato
mesa	— table	tortilla de huevos	— omelet
naranjas	— oranges	uvas	— grapes
papas	— potatoes	vaso	— glass
pastel	— pie	verdura	— greens
pavo	— turkey	zanahorias	— carrots
pepinos	— cucumbers		

3. Numbers — Números

31 treinta y uno	thirty-one	60 sesenta	sixty	90 noventa	ninety
40 cuarenta	forty	70 setenta	seventy	91 noventa y uno	ninety-one
50 cincuenta	fifty	80 ochenta	eighty	100 cien (ciento)	one hundred

4. Spanish names — Nombres hispanos   Nombres ingleses — English names

Beatriz	Héctor	Cheri	Darlene
Carmen	Irma	Cheryl	Dayl
Efraín	Julio	Cindy	Dean
Ester	Manuel	Connie	Dennis
Fernando	Marta	Cynthia	Diana
Gladys	Raúl	Daniel	Donald

5. Clothing — Ropa

bata	— robe	corbata	— necktie	pañuelo	— handkerchief
blusa	— blouse	chaqueta	— jacket	piyama	— pajamas
bufanda	— scarf	falda	— skirt	ropa interior	— underwear
calcetines	— socks	guantes	— gloves	sombrero	— hat
camisa	— shirt	impermeable	— raincoat	traje	— suit
cartera, bolso	— purse	medias	— hose	vestido	— dress
cinto, cinturón	— belt	pantalón	— pants, trousers	zapatos	— shoes

6. Useful expressions — Expresiones útiles

De mi medida	— my size	La ropa es muy cara	— clothing is very expensive.
La comida está deliciosa	— The food is delicious	Me gustan las frutas	— I like fruit

¿Necesita usar el baño?	— Do you need to use the restroom?	Un buen restaurante	— a good restaurant
No se olvide de dejar la propina	— Don't forget to leave a tip.	Un color claro	— a light color
Pasado mañana	— the day after tomorrow	Un color oscuro	— a dark color
		Un poco pesado	— a little bit heavy
		Un precio muy barato	— a very cheap price

7. Idiomatic expressions — Expresiones idiomáticas

A carta cabal	— thoroughly, fully	Hacer cola	— to stand in line
De memoria	— by heart	Sin querer	— unintentionally
Estar de luto	— to be in mourning	Valer la pena	— to be worth the trouble
Estar de moda	— to be popular, fashionable		

Trabajar to work

BILINGUAL PROJECT — PROYECTO BILINGUE

PREPARATORY EXERCISE 3 — EJERCICIO PREPARATORIO 3

When sending out statements it is better to itemize even if the fees have been explained before. On page 27 is an example of an itemized statement.

Put together a statement based on this model.

Cuando se envían los estados de cuenta, conviene explicar los servicios aun cuando los honorarios se hayan explicado antes. En la página siguiente se presenta un ejemplo de un estado de cuenta dado en detalle.

Haga un estado de cuenta siguiendo este modelo.

STATEMENT
ESTADO DE CUENTA

Frank L. Donalson, M.D.
210 Blue Bonnett
Keene, Texas 76059

Telephone (817) 641-7702

Mrs. Allan Miranda
100 Rosedale
Keene, Texas 76059

Receipt No. Recibo No.	Date Fecha	Professional Service Servicio profesional	Charge Monto		Paid Pagado		Balance Saldo	
1553	4/20	OC	25	00	25	00		00
1930	8/20	PE	32	00	10	00	22	00
2122	2/15	HC	40	00		00	40	00

Pay last amount in this column   62   00
Pague la última cantidad de esta columna

OC Office Call — Visita consult.   OS Office Surgery — Cirugía consult.
HC House Call — Visita hogar   HS Hospital Surgery — Cirugía hosp.
HOSP Hospital Care — Cuidado hosp. PE Physical Exam. — Examen físico
L Laboratory — Laboratorio   XR X-Ray — Radiografía

Other itemized charges — Otros cobros detallados

INS — Insurance — Seguros
OB — Obstetrical Care — Cuidado obstétrico
PAP — Papanicolaou Test — Examen Papanicolaou

EKG — Electrocardiogram — Electrocardiograma
I — Inyection — Inyección
NC — No charge — Sin cobro

EXERCISES — EJERCICIOS

(Students learning Spanish — Estudiantes de Español)

A. Fill in the blanks with the correct form of the verb ir.

1. Yo _____ al mercado.
2. Tú _____ al hospital.
3. El doctor _____ a la sala de operaciones
4. Los pacientes _____ a sus cuartos.
5. Julio y Ernesto _____ a la enfermería.
6. Los deportistas _____ al estudio.
7. Luis y yo _____ a la universidad.
8. Gloria _____ a la tienda.
9. Nosotros _____ al laboratorio.
10. La señora _____ a la sala de maternidad.

B. Translate into Spanish.

1. I am going to the store to buy a suit. ....
2. We have a few uniforms. ....
3. We eat at the restaurant. ....
4. The food is delicious. ....
5. Where do you work? ....

C. Fill in the blanks with the correct form of the verb tener.

1. Yo _____ un fuerte dolor de cabeza.
2. Tú _____ un resfrío.
3. Mi hermano _____ muchos trajes.
4. Los laboratoristas _____ poco trabajo.
5. Gabriel y yo _____ bastantes amigos.

D. Describe your favorite dish.

....
....

E. Answer in complete Spanish.

1. ¿Adónde va usted los fines de semana? ....
2. ¿Cuándo recibió usted su último estado de cuenta? ....
3. ¿De qué color es su uniforme? ....
4. ¿Cuál es su restaurante favorito? ....
5. ¿Dónde compra usted su ropa? .. ..

EJERCICIOS — EXERCISES

(Estudiantes de inglés — Students learning English)

A. Llene el espacio vacío con la preposición que falta.

1. When are you _____?
2. He is coming _____ me.
3. The house is _____ brick.
4. The doctor is _____ the hospital.

5. The money is _____ the drawer.
6. The flower is _____ the vase.
7. I am going _____ Spain.

8. John asks _____ you.
9. María lives _____ this country.
10. We are going _____ Joe's house.

B. Coloque el artículo (a, an, the) correspondiente en el espacio vacío — si se necesita.

1. He needs _____ operation.
2. _____ Mr. Johnston is a good physician.
3. I like _____ flowers.
4. He has _____ apple.
5. This book is for _____ Mr. Smith.

6. This is _____ watch.
7. We like _____ sports.
8. _____ nurse is intelligent.
9. They are _____ patients.
10. You are _____ doctor.

C. Haga una lista en inglés de sus platillos favoritos.

. . . .

. . . .

D. Haga una lista de las cuentas que le toca pagar a usted a fin de mes.

. . . .

. . . .

E. Conteste estas preguntas en inglés.

1. Who is your father? . . . .
2. Where do you work? . . . .
3. Where are you from? . . . .
4. Where is the hospital? . . . .
5. Who is your doctor? . . . .

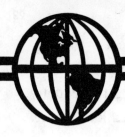

HOURS AND DATES
HORAS Y FECHAS

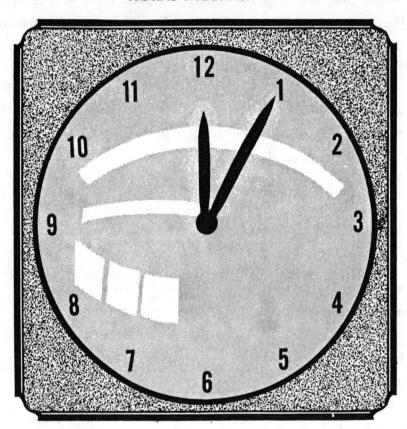

VOCABULARY — VOCABULARIO

A. Medical — Médico

ataque	— attack	maligno	— malignant
benigno	— benign	nervioso (a)	— nervous
hinchado (a)	— swollen, swelled	seco (a)	— dry, dried
hipo	— hiccup	sudor	— sweat
lucidez	— sanity	urticaria	— hives

B. General

acá, aquí	— here	durar	— to last
alquilar	— to rent	mes	— month
allá	— there	Nochebuena	— Christmas Eve
año	— year	próximo	— next
año bisiesto	— leap year	semana	— week
Año Nuevo	— New Year	sol	— sun
día de fiesta,		tarde	— late
día feriado	— holiday	temprano	— early
Día de Navidad	— Christmas Day		

CONVERSATION — CONVERSACION

A. Mercedes and Alvaro meet Sandy in the cafeteria.

Mercedes y Alvaro se encuentran con Sandy en la cafetería.

Sandy — How are you, guys?

¿Cómo están, muchachos?

Alvaro — Very well, thank you. How are you, Sandy?

Bien, gracias. ¿Cómo estás tú, Sandy?

Sandy — Fine. ¿Cómo estás, Mercedes?

Muy bien. How are you, Mercedes?

Mercedes — Muy bien, Sandy; lamento no saber inglés como Alvaro, pero tú estás mejorando mucho tu español.

Very well, Sandy; I'm sorry I don't know English as well as Alvaro, but you're doing fine in Spanish.

Sandy — I am trying my best. Alvaro, what time is it?

Me estoy esforzando lo más que puedo. Alvaro, ¿qué hora es?

Alvaro — It's seven forty-five.

Son las siete y cuarenta y cinco.

Sandy — It's late. I have a class at eight.

Es tarde. Tengo una clase a las ocho.

Mercedes — ¿A qué hora te acuestas, Sandy?

At what time do you go to bed, Sandy?

Sandy — Usually I go to bed at eleven and get up at six.

Por lo general me acuesto a las once y me levanto a las seis.

Alvaro — I usually go to bed at the same time, too.

Yo también me acuesto por lo general a la misma hora.

Mercedes — Y yo también.

Me too.

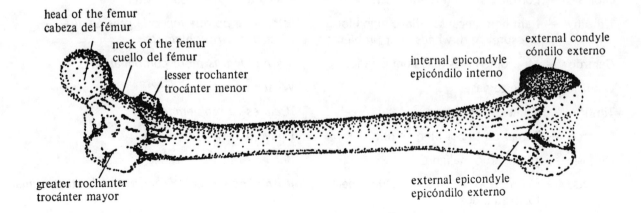

head of the femur
cabeza del fémur

neck of the femur
cuello del fémur

lesser trochanter
trocánter menor

internal epicondyle
epicóndilo interno

external condyle
cóndilo externo

greater trochanter
trocánter mayor

external epicondyle
epicóndilo externo

GRAMMATICAL HINTS — APUNTES GRAMATICALES

A. Preguntas con **or** - o; **what** - qué; **who** - quién (qué); **whose** - de quién.

1. Or se usa por lo general en medio de dos objetos.
   e.g. Is this a hospital **or** a clinic?

2. What se usa con expresiones tanto en singular como en plural.
   e.g. **What** is in the box? (¿Qué hay en la caja?)
   What are those medicines? (¿Qué clase de medicinas son esas?)

3. Who se refiere a una o más personas.
   e.g. **Who** is he?, **Who** are they?, (¿Quién es él?, ¿quiénes son ellas?)

4. Whose es la forma posesiva de **who.**
   e.g. **Whose** brother is he? (¿De quién es hermano él?)

B. ¿Qué hora es?   —   What time is it?

To express time in Spanish, the definite article is used to introduce the hour. When it is one o'clock, the verb and article are singular. When the hour is more than one, the verb and article are plural.

Es la una y media	— It is one-thirty.	Son las ocho y cinco	— It is five after eight.
Son las dos menos cuarto	— It is is quarter to two.	Son las doce en punto	— It is twelve sharp.

C. Cuando se da la hora en inglés se responde siempre en singular.
   It is   (It's)_____
   e.g. It's ten minutes after nine — Son las nueve y diez.

CONVERSATION — CONVERSACION (Cont.)

B. Timothy, Gerardo and Dionisio talk in the hospital room about their problems.

Gerardo, Timothy y Dionisio conversan acerca de sus problemas en su cuarto del **hospital.**

Gerardo — ¿Por qué están ustedes aquí?

¿Why are you here?

Dionisio — Porque tengo un fuerte resfriado.

Because I have a bad cold.

Timothy — I am here because I have high blood pressure. And, what's your problem?

Estoy aquí porque tengo la presión alta. ¿Y cuál es tu problema?

Gerardo — Mi problema es más complicado.

My problem is more complicated.

Dionisio — ¿Qué te pasa?

What's wrong with you?

Timothy — What's wrong?

¿Cuál es tu problema?

Gerardo — Tengo un tumor bien grande.

I have a very large tumor.

Dionisio — ¿Benigno o maligno?

Benign or malignant?

Gerardo — No se sabe todavía. Hay que esperar los resultados.

It isn't known yet. We must wait for the results.

Timothy — I hope your tumor is benign.

Espero que el tumor sea benigno.

Dionisio — Yo también. ¿Cuándo te operan?

Me too. When is the operation?

Gerardo — El martes a las siete.

Tuesday at seven.

Timothy — Good luck.

Buena suerte.

GRAMMATICAL HINTS — APUNTES GRAMATICALES (Cont.)

D. In the former lessons we have covered the present indicative of four irregular verbs: **estar, ser, ir, tener.**

The present indicative of the regular verbs in the first conjugation has the following endings: **-o, -as, -a, -amos, -an.**

yo	trabaj**o**	—	I work
tú	trabaj**as**	—	you (fam. sing.) work
él, ella, usted	trabaj**a**	—	he, she, works; you (for. sing) work; (it works: trabaja).
nosotros (as)	trabaj**amos**	—	we work
ellos, ellas, ustedes	trabaj**an**	—	they, you (for, plur.) work

E. Mientras que en español hay tres clases de verbos (las terminaciones verbales **ar, er, ir**), en inglés solamente hay una (señalada mediante la preposición **to**), y por lo tanto hay menos complicaciones en la conjugación de los verbos ingleses.

e.g. I work in the hospital — trabajo en el hospital.

She eats in the cafeteria — ella come en la cafetería.

CONVERSATION — CONVERSACION (Cont.)

C. The English teacher asks his students some questions.

El profesor de inglés les hace algunas preguntas a sus estudiantes.

Professor — Esteban, what is today's date?

Esteban, ¿cuál es la fecha de hoy?

Esteban — Today is October 11.

Hoy es el once de octubre.

Professor — Good! Consuelo, what are the seasons of the year?

¡Muy bien!. Consuelo, ¿cuáles son las estaciones del año?

Consuelo — Professor, the seasons of the year are: spring, summer, autumn, and winter.

Profesor, las estaciones del año son: la primavera, el verano, el otoño y el invierno.

Professor — All right. What are the days of the week? Let's see, Felipe.

Bien. ¿Cuáles son los días de la semana? Vamos a ver, Felipe.

Felipe — No los sé todos.

I don't know them all.

Professor — In English.

En inglés.

Felipe — I don't know them all.

No los sé todos.

Professor — Rafael, the same question.

Rafael, la misma pregunta.

Rafael — The days of the week are: Sunday, Monday, Tuesday, Wednesday, Thursday, Friday, and Saturday.

Los días de la semana son: el domingo, el lunes, el martes, el miércoles, el jueves, el viernes y el sábado.

Professor — Excellent. Ruth, what are the months of the year?

Excelente. Ruth, ¿cuáles son los meses del año?

Ruth — Los meses del año son ...

The months of the year are ...

Professor — In English.

En inglés.

Ruth	— January, February, March, April, May, June, July, August, September, October, November, December.	*Enero, febrero, marzo, abril, mayo, junio, julio, agosto, septiembre (or setiembre), octubre, noviembre, diciembre.*
Professor	— Good. Carlos, what day of the week do you like best?	*Bien. Carlos, ¿qué día de la semana le gusta a usted más?*
Carlos	— I like Sundays because we don't have classes.	*Me gustan los domingos porque no tenemos clases.*
Professor	— You're right. Eunice, What time is it?	*Tiene razón. Eunice, ¿qué hora es?*
Eunice	— Exactly two-thirty.	*Exactamente las dos y treinta.*
Professor	— Then it's time to finish. We are dismissed.	*Entonces es tiempo de terminar. Podemos salir del aula.*

ADDITIONAL INFORMATION — INFORMACION ADICIONAL

1. Days of the week — Días de la semana

domingo	— Sunday	jueves	— Thursday
lunes	— Monday	viernes	— Friday
martes	— Tuesday	sábado	— Saturday
miércoles	— Wednesday		

2. Months of the year — Meses del año

enero	— January	mayo	— May	septiembre	— September
febrero	— February	junio	— June	octubre	— October
marzo	— March	julio	— July	noviembre	— November
abril	— April	agosto	— August	diciembre	— December

3. Seasons of the year — Estaciones del año

primavera	— spring	otoño	— autumn
verano	— summer	invierno	— winter

4. Spanish names — Nombres hispanos   Nombres ingleses — English names

Alvaro	Felipe	Debbie	Dorothy
Carlos	Flor	Dee	Douglas
Consuelo	Gilberto	Denise	Dwight
Esmeralda	Hilda	Diane	Earl
Esteban	Humberto	Donna	Edward
Eunice	Mercedes	Doris	Eric

5. Numbers — Números

101	ciento uno — a hundred and one	600	seiscientos — six hundred
102	ciento dos — a hundred and two	700	setecientos — seven hundred
110	ciento diez — a hundred and ten	800	ochocientos — eight hundred
200	doscientos — two hundred	900	novecientos — nine hundred
300	trescientos — three hundred	1,000	mil — one thousand
400	cuatrocientos — four hundred	10,000	diez mil — ten thousand
500	quinientos — five hundred	100,000	cien mil — one hundred thousand
		1,000,000	un millón — one million

6. Useful expressions — Expresiones útiles

¿Qué día es hoy?	— What day is today?
Hoy es martes	— Today is Tuesday.
Tengo que llegar a tiempo	— I have to be on time.
¿Anda bien ese reloj?	— Is that clock right?
¿Cuánto se demora?	— How long does it take?
¿Pudiera decirme qué hora es?	— Could you tell me what time it is?
¿Cuál es la mejor hora para venir?	— When is the best time to come?
¿Dentro de cuánto tiempo?	— How soon?
Espere un momento	— Wait a minute.
Tan pronto como sea posible	— As soon as possible
Según mi reloj	— According to my watch
Mi reloj se atrasa	— My watch is slow.
Mi reloj se adelanta	— My watch is fast.
¿Adónde va usted?	— Where are you going?
Debo irme	— I must go.

7. Idioms — Modismos

Al mismo tiempo	— at the same time
A su debido tiempo	— in due time
¿Cuál es la fecha? ¿A cómo estamos?	— What's the date?
El avión llegó tarde	— The plane arrived late
En poco tiempo	— in a short time
Por fin, por última vez	— finally, for the last time
Por la noche	— at night, in the evening
Por la tarde	— In the afternoon
Por primera vez	— for the first time
¿Qué hora es?	— What time is it?
Tarde o temprano	— sooner or later
Todavía no	— not yet

8. Some sports — Algunos deportes

atletismo	— athletics	fútbol	— soccer, football
baloncesto	— basketball	golf	— golf
béisbol	— baseball	jai alai	— jai alai
boxeo	— boxing	levantamiento de pesas	— weight lifting
caminatas	— hiking	lucha libre	— wrestling
ciclismo	— bicycling	natación	— swimming
deportes	— sports	pesca	— fishing
equitación	— horseback riding, horsemanship	tenis	— tennis
esquí acuático	— water skiing	trote	— jogging
esquí en la nieve	— snow skiing	volibol	— volleyball

BILINGUAL PROJECT — PROYECTO BILINGUE

PREPARATORY EXERCISE 4 — EJERCICIO PREPARATORIO 4

A medical history consists of pertinent information obtained from a patient.

La historia médica es la información pertinente que se obtiene del paciente.

Make your own patient history by giving the necessary information.

Haga su propia historia médica dando la información necesaria.

MEDICAL HISTORY OUTLINE
GUIA PARA UNA HISTORIA MEDICA

PATIENT
PACIENTE _____

ADDRESS
DIRECCION _____

HISTORY
HISTORIA

Order of Recording
Orden de registro

1. Chief Complaint
   Síntoma principal
2. History of Present
   Illness
   Historia de la enfer-
   medad actual
3. History of Past
   Illness
   Historia de enfer-
   medades anteriores
   a) Child
      Niño
   b) Adult
      Adulto
   c) Operations
      Operaciones
   d) Injuries
      Heridas
4. Family History
   Historia de la familia
5. Social History
   Historia social
6. Systemic Review
   Repaso sistemático
   a) General — General
   b) Skin — Piel
   c) Head — Cabeza, Eyes — Ojos, Ears — Orejas,
      Nose — Nariz, Throat — Garganta
   d) Neck — Cuello
   e) Respiratory — Respiratorio
   f) Cardiovascular — Cardiovascular
   g) Gastrointestinal — Gastrointestinal
   h) Genitourinary — Genitourinario
   i) Gynecological — Ginecológico
   j) Locomotor — Locomotor
   k) Neuropsychiatric — Neurosiquiátrico
7. Signature
   Firma

EXERCISES — EJERCICIOS

(Students learning Spanish — Estudiantes de español)

A. Translate the following sentences into Spanish.

1. It is one-thirty. ....

2. I work at the hospital. ....

3. It is three-twenty-five. ....

4. We are students. ....

5. It is late. ....

B. Fill in the blanks with the correct form of the verb in the present indicative.

1. El doctor _____ en el hospital. (trabajar)

2. La enfermera _____ un uniforme nuevo. (comprar)

3. El paciente _____ la cuenta. (pagar)

4. Los familiares _____ al muerto. (llorar)

5. Los farmacéuticos _____ la receta. (preparar)

6. Tú _____ en la universidad. (estudiar)

7. Yo _____ la lección. (explicar)

8. Juan y yo _____ el carro. (lavar)

9. Juan _____ en la piscina. (nadar)

C. Write six complete sentences with the idioms you already know.

1. ....   4. ....

2. ....   5. ....

3. ....   6. ....

D. Answer with a complete sentence in Spanish.

1. ¿Qué días trabaja usted? ....

2. ¿Qué días tiene libres? ....

3. ¿Cuáles son los meses de invierno? ¿de verano? ....

4. ¿Cuál es la fecha de hoy? ....

5. ¿Qué hora es? ....

E. Make up a schedule of a typical working day.

Helping phrases — Frases que ayudan

I get up	— me levanto.	I get dressed	— me visto.
I go to bed	— me acuesto.	I eat breakfast	— desayuno.
I go to work	— voy al trabajo.	I study	— estudio.
I take a bath	— me baño.	I brush my teeth	— me lavo los dientes.
I shave myself	— me afeito.	I eat dinner	— ceno.
I comb my hair	— me peino.	I eat lunch	— almuerzo.

I go to the store	— voy a la tienda.	I take a nap	— duermo una siesta.
I greet my family	— saludo a mi familia.	I take care of a	— cuido a un
I meet some friends	— me encuentro con	patient	paciente.
	unos amigos.	I visit the doctor	— visito al doctor.
I write a letter	— escribo una carta.	I go to the hospital	— voy al hospital.
I see my family	— veo a mi familia.		

EJERCICIOS — EXERCISES

(Estudiantes de inglés — Students learning English)

A. Confeccione un programa de un día típico de trabajo. (Vea la lista de frases que ayudan en la pág. 37).

B. Haga seis preguntas usando or, what, who, y whose.

1. . . . .   4. . . . .

2. . . . .   5. . . . .

3. . . . .   6. . . . .

C. Traduzca las siguientes oraciones al inglés.

1. Son las nueve y media. . . . .

2. Me acuesto y me levanto temprano. . . . .

3. ¿Qué hora es? . . . .

4. La estación más hermosa es la primavera. . . . .
. . . .

5. No tenemos clases los sábados. . . . .
. . . .

D. Conteste en inglés.

1. What days do you work? . . . .

2. What time is it? . . . .

3. When do you go to school? . . . .

4. What is your favorite sport? . . . .

5. What is your favorite subject at the university? . . . .

E. Escriba seis oraciones con las expresiones idiomáticas que ya sabe.

1. . . . .   4. . . . .

2. . . . .   5. . . . .

3. . . . .   6. . . . .

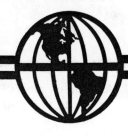

THE ANATOMY CLASS
LA CLASE DE ANATOMIA

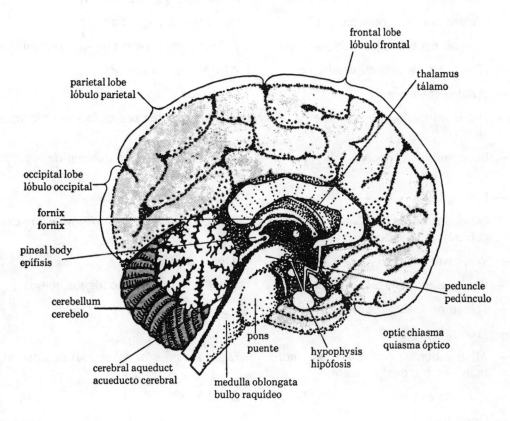

frontal lobe
lóbulo frontal

thalamus
tálamo

parietal lobe
lóbulo parietal

occipital lobe
lóbulo occipital

fornix
fornix

pineal body
epífisis

peduncle
pedúnculo

cerebellum
cerebelo

optic chiasma
quiasma óptico

pons
puente

hypophysis
hipófosis

cerebral aqueduct
acueducto cerebral

medulla oblongata
bulbo raquídeo

VOCABULARY — VOCABULARIO

A. Medical — Médico

brazo	— arm	corazón	— heart	órgano	— organ
células	— cells	cuerpo	— body	oxígeno	— oxygen
cerebro	— brain	hueso	— bone	pulmón	— lung
circulación	— circulation	muerte	— death	sangre	— blood

B. General

a través	— through	importante	— important
administrar	— to administer	manar	— to pour forth
alimento	— food	morir	— to die
apenas	— just about, about	muchachas	— girls
aunque	— although	muchachos	— boys
capaz	— able	mujer	— woman
dejar de, parar	— to stop	perjudicar	— to damage
diversos (as)	— several, various	saber	— to know
funcionar	— to function	siempre	— always, ever
hombre	— man	sin	— without

CONVERSATION — CONVERSACION

A. William meets Rose and Delia on the campus of the university at which they are studying.

Guillermo se encuentra con Rose y Delia en el campo de la Universidad donde están estudiando.

William	— Hello, Rose and Delia, how are you?	*Hola, Rose y Delia, ¿cómo están?*
Rose	— We are fine, and how are you?	*Estamos bien, ¿y cómo estás tú?*
William	— I am all right, but just a bit worried.	*Yo estoy bien, pero un poco preocupado.*
Delia	— ¿Por qué estás preocupado?	*Why are you worried?*
William	— What is she saying?	*¿Qué dice ella?*
Rose	— She is wondering why you are worried.	*Ella quiere saber por qué estás preocupado.*
William	— Because I have a very hard anatomy exam today.	*Porque hoy tengo un examen de anatomía muy difícil.*
Rose	— Porque tiene...	*Because he has...*
Delia	— Entiendo. Ahora pregúntale qué cubrirán en el examen.	*I understand. Now ask him what the exam will cover.*
Rose	— What will it cover?	*¿Qué cubrirá?*
William	— We have to know all the bones.	*Tenemos que saber todos los huesos.*
Rose	— Tienen que saber todos los huesos.	
Delia	— ¿Todos los huesos?	
William	— All the bones. And there are more than two hundred of them.	*Todos los huesos. Y hay más de doscientos.*
Delia	— Buena suerte.	*Good luck.*
Rose	— Good luck.	
William	— Thank you. I need it.	*Gracias. La necesito.*

GRAMMATICAL HINTS — APUNTES GRAMATICALES

A. The thing liked is always the **subject** of the verb **gustar,** whereas in English the thing liked is always the **object** of **to like.**

When the **subject** is singular, the form of the verb is singular.
When the **subject** of the verb is plural, the form is plural.

> Me gusta la universidad (subject). — I like the university (object).
> Te gusta la cafetería. — you like the cafeteria.
> Le gusta el deporte. — he likes sports.
> Nos gusta el hospital. — we like the hospital.
> Les gusta el mercado. — they like the market.
> Me gust**an las** flor**es.** — I like flowers.
> Nos gust**an los** deport**es.** — we like sports.

B. Some-Any (alguno y ninguno)

1. Some se usa en ocasiones afirmativas.
   e.g. I have some money — Tengo algún dinero.

2. Any se usa en ocasiones negativas.
   e.g. I don't have any good medicine — no tengo ninguna medicina buena.

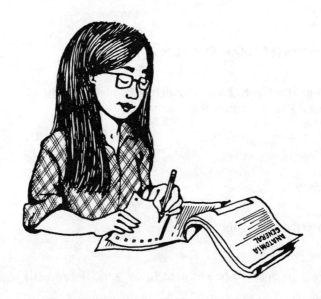

CONVERSATION — CONVERSACION (Cont.)

B. Modesta, Esperanza and Gina —an American student— are talking before the anatomy class begins.

Modesta, Esperanza y Gina —una estudiante norteamericana— hablan antes de que comience la clase de anatomía.

Gina — Dr. Duarte is in the hall talking with another professor.

El Dr. Duarte está en el pasillo hablando con otro profesor.

Modesta — Y parece que trae los exámenes en la mano.

And it looks like he is bringing the exams with him.

Esperanza — ¿Tienes miedo? Es tan sólo un examen.

Are you afraid? It's only a test.

Gina — It's only a test.

(After the test.)

(*Después del examen*).

Modesta — Te apuesto a que no nos fue muy bien.

I'll bet you we didn't do too well.

Esperanza — ¿Por qué crees eso?

Why do you think so?

Gina — Why?

Modesta — Era muy largo. Más de 150 puntos.

It was a very long one. More than 150 points.

Gina — But we knew all the answers.

Pero nosotras sabíamos todas las respuestas.

Modesta — No todas. Había algunas preguntas que no estaban muy claras.

Not all of them. There were some questions that weren't very clear.

Gina	—	They weren't clear, even to me.	*No estaban claras, aun para mí.*
Esperanza	—	Déjate de tonterías, Modesta. Te apuesto a que a todas nos fue bien.	*Stop being silly, I'll bet that we all did well.*
Modesta	—	Así lo espero.	*I hope so.*
Gina	—	Me too.	*Yo también.*

GRAMMATICAL HINTS — APUNTES GRAMATICALES (Cont.)

C. Saber

The verb **saber** means in Spanish to have knowledge of facts, or just plainly to know.
The verb **saber** conjugates in the following manner:

yo	sé	I know
tú	sabes	you (fam. sing.) know
él	sabe	he knows
nosotros	sabemos	we know
ellos	saben	they know

En inglés hay un solo verbo para **saber** y **conocer:** to know.

D. Conocer

The verb **conocer** means in Spanish to know or to be acquainted with persons, places, etc.

The verb **conocer** conjugates in the following manner: conozco, conoces, conoce, conocemos, conocen.

E. The conjugation of all regular verbs ending in **er** and **ir** follows this pattern:
Comer: como, comes, come, comemos, comen
Vivir: vivo, vives, vive, vivimos, viven

F. Como ya se ha notado las contracciones se usan más en inglés que en español. Las contracciones del verbo con el pronombre se usan generalmente en conversaciones. Un apóstrofe (') reemplaza la letra omitida.
No se usan contracciones en la forma interrogativa.
e.g. Are you a professor? — ¿Es usted profesor?
Yes, I'm a professor and you're a student — Sí, yo soy profesor y usted es un estudiante.

IN THE ANATOMY CLASS — EN LA CLASE DE ANATOMIA

In the class of anatomy and physiology the professor starts his lecture this way:

The heart is the most important organ of the human body because it maintains life. The heart is important to the life of men and animals because it regulates the circulation of blood throughout the body. By means of the blood that circulates through the body oxygen and food are supplied to the diverse cells of the body. If the heart stops beating the brain is damaged forever. Man lives while his heart is beating, if it stops man dies. Man is capable of living without an arm, without a lung, or a hand, but not without a heart.

Answer the following questions:

1. What is the most important part of the body?

2. Why is blood circulation so important?

3. Why is oxygen necessary?

4. What happens when the heart stops beating?

5. Why can a man live without a lung but not without his heart?

En la clase de anatomía y fisiología el profesor comienza su disertación de esta manera:

El corazón es el órgano más importante del cuerpo humano porque conserva la vida. El corazón es importante en la vida del hombre porque regula la circulación de la sangre a través de todo el cuerpo. Por la circulación de la sangre por el cuerpo el oxígeno y el alimento son llevados a las diversas células del cuerpo. Si el corazón deja de trabajar el cerebro se daña para siempre; si se para, el hombre muere. El hombre es capaz de vivir sin un brazo, un pulmón o una mano, pero no sin el corazón.

Conteste a las preguntas siguientes:

¿Cuál es la parte más importante del cuerpo?

¿Por qué es la circulación de la sangre tan importante?

¿Por qué es necesario el oxígeno?

¿Qué sucede cuando el corazón se para?

¿Por qué puede un hombre vivir sin un pulmón pero no sin el corazón?

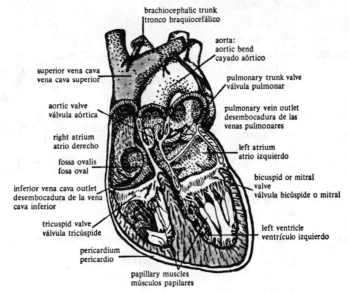

brachiocephalic trunk
tronco braquiocefálico

aorta:
aortic bend
cayado aórtico

superior vena cava
vena cava superior

pulmonary trunk valve
válvula pulmonar

aortic valve
válvula aórtica

pulmonary vein outlet
desembocadura de las
venas pulmonares

right atrium
atrio derecho

fossa ovalis
fosa oval

left atrium
atrio izquierdo

inferior vena cava outlet
desembocadura de la vena
cava inferior

bicuspid or mitral
valve
válvula bicúspide o mitral

tricuspid valve
válvula tricúspide

left ventricle
ventrículo izquierdo

pericardium
pericardio

papillary muscles
músculos papilares

ADDITIONAL INFORMATION — INFORMACION ADICIONAL

1. Parts of the body — Partes del cuerpo

antebrazo	— forearm	cintura	— waist
axila, el sobaco	— armpit	codo	— elbow
cadera	— hip	costilla	— rib

dedos	— fingers
dedos del pie	— toes
espalda	— back
espinilla	— shin
estómago	— stomach
hombro	— shoulder
juanete	— bunion
mano	— hand
muñeca	— wrist
muslo	— thigh
nuca	— nape of the neck
pecho	— chest
pie	— foot
rabadilla	— coccyx
rodilla	— knee
tobillo	— ankle

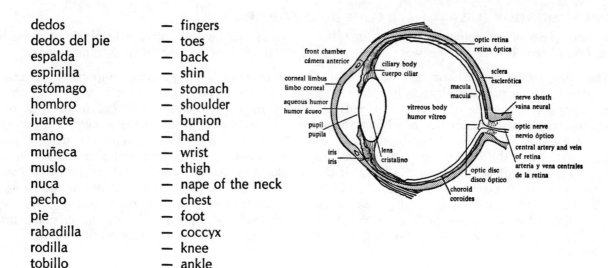

2. Ordinal Numbers   Números ordinales

primero	— first
segundo	— second
tercero	— third
cuarto	— fourth
quinto	— fifth

sexto	— sixth
séptimo	— seventh
octavo	— eighth
noveno	— ninth
décimo	— tenth

3. Some of the most important languages of the world — Algunas de las lenguas más importantes del mundo.

alemán	— German
árabe	— Arabic
chino	— Chinese
español, castellano	— Spanish
francés	— French
griego	— Greek
hindú	— Hindi
inglés	— English
italiano	— Italian
japonés	— Japanese
persa, iraní	— Persian, Iranian
portugués	— Portuguese
rumano	— Rumanian
ruso	— Russian

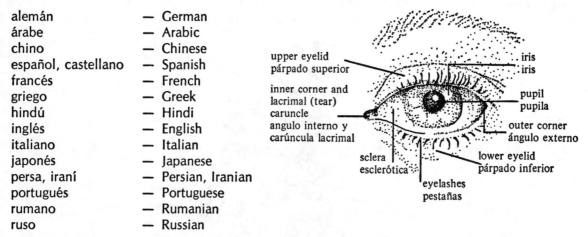

4. Spanish names — Nombres hispanos   Nombres ingleses — English names

David	Olga	Allan	Oscar
Doris	Oscar	David	Reuben
Félix	Remigio	Don	Richard
Hernando	Rodrigo	Hope	Robert
Moisés	Rosaura	Mary	Sandy
Mónica	Rubén	Moses	Susy
Nubia	Sandra	Nancy	Tony

5. Some college majors — Algunas especialidades universitarias

administración de empresas	— business administration	física	— physics
agricultura	— agriculture	fotografía	— photography
arte	— art	geografía	— geography
astronomía	— astronomy	geología	— geology
bibliotecología, biblioteconomía	— library science	historia	— history
		lenguas modernas	— modern languages
biología	— biology	literatura	— literature
canto	— singing	magisterio	— teaching
comercio	— business	matemáticas	— mathematics
comunicación	— communication	medicina	— medicine
contabilidad	— accounting	microbiología	— microbiology
derecho	— law	ministerio	— ministry
economía doméstica	— home economics	música	— music
educación, pedagogía	— education	periodismo	— journalism
educación física	— physical education	química	— chemistry
educación industrial	— industrial education	secretariado	— secretarial science
enfermería	— nursing	sicología	— psychology
		sociología	— sociology

6. Idiomatic expressions — Expresiones idiomáticas

a fin de cuentas	— in the final analysis	llevarse una sorpresa	— to be surprised
a más tardar	— at the latest	no poder con	— not to be able to do...
al entrar	— on entering		
de modo que	— so (that)	ocuparse de	— to concern oneself about, to take care of
echar a perder	— to ruin, to spoil		
fracasar en la materia	— to fail or "flunk" the subject		
		pedir prestado	— to borrow
hacerse el dueño	— to become the master	sacar buenas notas o calificaciones	— to get good grades
ir al grano	— to get to the point		

7. Useful expressions — Expresiones útiles

la medicina es difícil	— medicine is hard.	¿Qué piensa hacer Ud. esta noche?	— what are you planning to do tonight?
el profesor vendrá mañana	— the professor will come tomorrow.		
despiértame temprano, por favor	— call me early, please.	tengan cuidado	— be careful.
¿Cuántas materias está tomando este trimestre?	— how many subjects are you taking this quarter?	voy a estudiar en seguida	— I am going to study right away.
		tenemos laboratorio dos veces por semana	— we have lab twice a week.
salir bien	— to receive a passing grade		
cuesta como cinco dólares la libra	— it costs about five dollars per pound.	dar clases	— to teach
		tener éxito	— to be successful
se me malogró el carro	— my car broke down.	¿Qué quiere decir con eso?	— what do you mean by that?
no tenemos clases los domingos	— we don't have classes on Sundays.		

BILINGUAL PROJECT — PROYECTO BILINGUE

PREPARATORY EXERCISE 5 — EJERCICIO PREPARATORIO 5

Professor Martin asks his students to transcribe a hospital situation while taking into consideration the following words and expressions.

El Profesor Martin les pide a los alumnos que transcriban una situación que haya ocurrido en el hospital teniendo en consideración las siguientes palabras y expresiones.

WORDS AND EXPRESSIONS — PALABRAS Y EXPRESIONES

arthritis	— artritis	hiccup	— hipo
astigmatism	— astigmatismo	neuralgia	— neuralgia
caffeine	— cafeína	pharmacist	— farmacéutico
diabetes	— diabetes	pulmonary	— pulmonar
eczema	— eczema	symptoms?	— síntomas?
I feel bad	— me siento mal.	Don't worry about it	— no se preocupe de eso.
The situation is serious	— la situación es grave.	This medicine contains ...	— Esta medicina contiene ...
The operation is necessary	— la operación es necesaria.	Did you notice the...	— ¿Notó los...

NAME — NOMBRE ....

ADDRESS — DIRECCION ....

SITUATION — SITUACION ....

....

....

....

REPORT — INFORME ....

EXERCISES — EJERCICIOS

(Students learning Spanish — Estudiantes de español)

A. Translate into Spanish.

1. The nurse likes her work. ....

2. We like swimming. ....

3. The heart is a very important organ. ....

4. I have two classes today, including the anatomy class. ....
   ....

5. There are over two hundred bones in the human body. ....
   ....

B. Fill in the blank with the appropriate form of the words in parentheses.

1. ¿Cómo _____ Ud. hoy? (están, estamos, está)

2. Los pacientes _____ mucha agua. (beben, bebe, bebes)

3. Ella _____ enfermera. (está, es, son)

4. La enfermera _____ la ventana. (abrir, abrimos, abre)

5. Ellos _____ el hospital. (conocen, conozco, conocemos)

C. Answer in Spanish.

1. ¿Por qué es importante la clase de anatomía? ....

2. ¿Cuál es la diferencia entre la anatomía y la fisiología? ....

3. ¿Qué lengua hablan en Suiza? ....

4. ¿Cuántas clases tiene usted los martes? ....

5. Mencione cinco órganos del cuerpo ....

(For Spanish and English students — Estudiantes de español e inglés)

D. Make a list of the requirements needed for your major in college. For instance, an associate degree in Office Administration with emphasis on training as a bilingual secretary requires the following subjects:

Haga una lista de los requisitos que se necesitan para su especialización. Por ejemplo, para recibir un diploma en la Administración de oficinas con énfasis en el Secretariado bilingüe se necesitan las siguientes materias:

Required courses:

Secretarial orientation
Personal development
Records Management
Reprographics
Office calculating machines
Machine transcription
Advanced typewriting
Professional typewriting
Business writing
Office procedures
Clerical accounting or Introduction to
   Accounting
The Bilingual Secretarial Training
Spanish Conversation
Hispanic-American Culture and Literature
The Development of Hispanic America and the
   Southwest
Special content vocabulary
Golden-Age literature
(Additional 20 hours with the major)

Materias requeridas:

Orientación para secretarias
Desarrollo personal
Administración de archivos
Reprografía
Máquinas calculadoras de oficina
Máquina de transcripción
Mecanografía avanzada
Mecanografía profesional
Redacción para el comercio
Prácticas de oficina
Contabilidad secretarial o Introducción a la
   contabilidad
Secretariado bilingüe
Conversación española
Cultura y literatura hispanoamericana
El desarrollo de la América Hispánica y el
   suroeste de los Estados Unidos
Vocabulario especial
Literatura del Siglo de Oro
(20 horas adicionales no incluidas entre las
   correspondientes a la especialización)

E. Write six complete sentences with some of the idiomatic expressions that you already know.

1. . . . .   4. . . . .

2. . . . .   5. . . . .

3. . . . .   6. . . . .

EJERCICIOS — EXERCISES

(Estudiantes de inglés — Students learning English)

A. Conteste cada pregunta en la forma afirmativa y negativa usando contracciones en las respuestas.

1. Are you a doctor? . . . .

2. Is she a nurse? . . . .

3. Are they pharmacists? . . . .

4. Are we patients? . . . .

5. Am I a student? . . . .

B. Conteste a las siguientes preguntas en inglés con oraciones completas.

1. How many bones are there in the human body? . . . .

2. Why is Chemistry important? . . . .

3. What is your favorite subject? . . . .

4. How many classes do you have on Thursdays? . . . .

5. What do you study? . . . .

C. Escriba seis oraciones con some y any.

1. . . . .   4. . . . .

2. . . . .   5. . . . .

3. . . . .   6. . . . .

D. Traduzca al inglés.

1. Me gustan las flores. . . . .

2. Hoy es lunes. . . . .

3. Hoy tenemos dos clases, pero mañana tenemos cuatro. . . . .

. . . .

4. El Inglés es una lengua muy importante . . . .

5. Los ojos están en la cara. . . . .

E. Escriba seis oraciones completas con las expresiones idiomáticas que usted ya conoce.

1. . . . .   4. . . . .

2. . . . .   5. . . . .

3. . . . .   6. . . . .

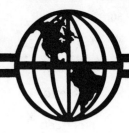

AT THE DOCTOR'S OFFICE
EN EL CONSULTORIO MEDICO

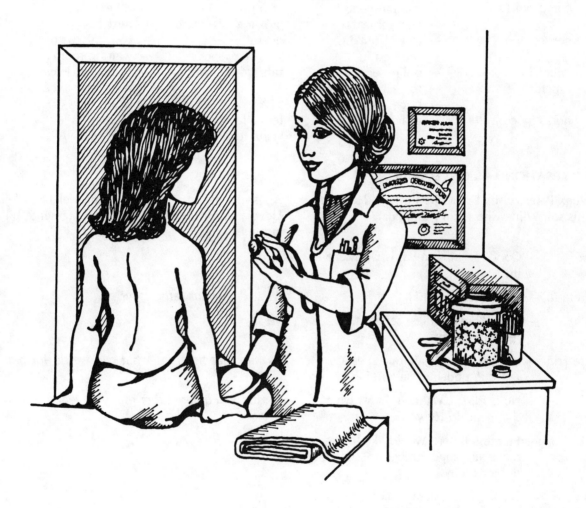

VOCABULARY — VOCABULARIO

A. Medical — Médico

ceguera	— blindness	jaqueca, migrania	— migraine
cicatriz	— scar	lesión	— lesion
cita	— appointment, date	moretón	— bruise
consultorio médico	— doctor's office	picazón	— itch
corte, cortada	— cut	sarampión	— measles
fiebre, calentura	— fever	sordomudo	— deaf-mute
fractura	— fracture		

B. General

abierto	— open	itinerario	— itinerary, schedule of travel
casi	— almost		
cerrado	— closed	juramento de Hipócrates	— Hippocratic oath
competente	— competent, reliable	oír	— to listen
compromisos	— commitments, engagements	otro (a)	— other
		próxima, siguiente	— next
conseguir	— to get, obtain, succeed in	querer	— to want, wish
		sala de espera	— waiting room
educado	— polite, educated	salir de vacaciones	— to take a, leave on, go on vacation
esperar	— to wait, wait for, hope, expect	silla	— chair
horas de consulta	— office hours	tenga la bondad	— please
		visita regular	— a regular visit

CONVERSATION — CONVERSACION

A. Alex Peters visits Dr. Mejía's office. He takes his son Willie who is fully bilingual.

Alejandro Peters visita la oficina del Dr. Mejía. Lleva a su hijo Willie que es perfectamente bilingüe.

Alex	— Good morning, miss, is Dr. Mejía in?	
Secretaria	— ¿Qué dice su papá?	*What does your father say?*
Willie	— Dice: "buenos días, señorita, ¿está el doctor?"	*He says ...*
Secretaria	— Buenos días, dígale que sí está; ¿en qué podemos servirle?	*Tell him that he is in; what can we do for him?*
Willie	— He is in; she wants to know what they can do for you.	*El está; ella quiere saber en qué pueden servirte.*
Alex	— Please tell her I would like to make an appointment to see the doctor today.	
Willie	— Dice que quisiera hacer una cita para ver al doctor hoy.	
Secretaria	— Dígale, por favor, que hoy no. Hoy tiene muchos compromisos. Tal vez mañana.	
Willie	— She says he has many appointments today. Perhaps tomorrow.	
Alex	— At what time tomorrow?	
Willie	— ¿Mañana a qué hora?	
Secretaria	— A las 9:30 a.m.	
Willie	— At 9:30 a.m.	

Alex	—	All right. We'll be here at that time.	
Willie	—	Está bien. Estaremos aquí a esa hora.	
Secretaria	—	Magnífico. ¿Cómo se llama tu padre?	*Good. What's your father's name?*
Willie	—	Se llama Alex Peters y yo me llamo Willie.	*His name is Alex Peters and I am Willie.*
Secretaria	—	Entonces los espero mañana.	
Alex	—	What did she say?	*¿Qué dijo?*
Willie	—	She said she'll be waiting for us tomorrow.	
Alex	—	Let's go then!	*Entonces vámonos.*
Willie	—	Adiós.	
Secretaria	—	Adiós.	
Alex	—	Good-by.	

GRAMMATICAL HINTS — APUNTES GRAMATICALES

A. Decir is an irregular verb. Its conjugation in the present indicative goes like this:

digo — I say
dices — you say
dice — he says
decimos — we say
dicen — they say
e.g. What do you say? — ¿Qué dice usted?

B. En inglés hay dos verbos que corresponden a **decir: say** y **tell.** El primero se usa para expresar, declarar, manifestar:
e.g. It's hard to say — Es difícil decir.
El segundo se usa para narrar, relatar o para informar:
e.g. I am going to tell you a story — Te voy a relatar una historia.

CONVERSATION — CONVERSACION (Cont.)

B. Lucho Martínez is feeling sick this morning, so he decides to visit Dr. Martin. After a long wait, the receptionist, Debbie Gil, ushers him into the doctor's office.

Lucho Martínez se siente mal esta mañana, por lo tanto decide visitar al Dr. Martin. Después de una larga espera, la recepcionista, Debbie Gil, lo lleva a la oficina del doctor.

Dr. Martin	—	Good morning, Mr. Martínez, how are you today?	
Debbie	—	El doctor quiere saber cómo está usted hoy.	*The doctor wants to know how you are today.*
Lucho	—	Estoy muy enfermo. Tengo un dolor en el pecho, me duele la cabeza y toso mucho.	

Debbie	—	He doesn't feel too well. He has a pain in his chest, he has a headache and is coughing a lot.
Dr. Martin	—	Let me examine you. Please sit down on this table.

Permítame examinarlo. Tenga la bondad de sentarse en esta mesa.

Debbie	—	El doctor lo va a examinar. Siéntese en esta mesa, por favor.
Lucho	—	Gracias. ¿Me quito la ropa?
Debbie	—	Should he take off his clothes?
Dr. Martin	—	Only his shirt.
Debbie	—	Solamente la camisa.

(Después de examinarlo, el doctor escribe una receta y se la entrega al paciente).*

*(After examining him, the doctor writes a prescription and gives it to the patient.)**

Dr. Martin	—	You have to take this prescription to a pharmacy; and before taking the medicine read the label.
Debbie	—	Tiene que presentar esta receta en una farmacia, y antes de tomar la medicina, lea la etiqueta.
Lucho	—	Gracias, señorita.

Thank you, miss.

Debbie	—	A sus órdenes.

You're welcome.

GRAMMATICAL HINTS — APUNTES GRAMATICALES (Cont.)

C. Possessive adjectives — Adjetivos posesivos

1. The possessive adjectives are:

Before a noun				After a noun		English
Sing.	**Pl.**	**Sing.**		**Pl.**		
		Mas.	**Fem.**	**Mas.**	**Fem.**	
mi	mis	mío	mía	míos	mías	— my
tu	tus	tuyo	tuya	tuyos	tuyas	— your (fam.)
su	sus	suyo	suya	suyos	suyas	— his, her, its, your (for., pl.), their

nuestro (a), nuestros (as), nuestro, nuestra nuestros, nuestras — our

2. Possessive adjectives agree in gender and number with the thing possessed.

e.g. mi casa — my house   la casa mía — my house
     mis casas — my houses   las casas mías — my houses

---

* The prescription said: take a pill every four hours. Take a tablespoonful of cough syrup before going to bed. Rub your chest with the ointment before going to bed.

* La receta decía: Tome una pastilla cada cuatro horas. Tome una cucharada de jarabe para la tos antes de acostarse. Póngase el ungüento en el pecho antes de acostarse, frotándolo bien.

3. Possessive adjectives which precede the noun are more frequently used than the ones that follow the noun. The definite article is used with the adjectives that follow the noun.
e.g. tus padres — your parents; **los** padres tuyos.

D. Possessive pronouns — Pronombres posesivos

1. The possessive pronouns are:

Singular		Plural		English
Mas.	**Fem.**	**Mas.**	**Fem.**	
el mío	la mía	los míos	las mías	— mine
el tuyo	la tuya	los tuyos	las tuyas	— yours (fam.)
el suyo	la suya	los suyos	las suyas	— his, hers, theirs, yours (for., pl.)
el nuestro	la nuestra	los nuestros	las nuestras	— ours

2. Possessive pronouns are used when the noun is omitted.
e.g. Tengo mi cuaderno — I have my notebook.
Tú tienes **el tuyo** — You have yours.

E. Otros posesivos — Other possessives

1. Además de todos los posesivos ya mencionados en esta lección, hay dos formas en inglés para indicar propiedad; una de ellas es usando la preposición **of** — **de**, tal como se usa en español.
e.g. the book **of** John — el libro **de** Juan

2. La otra forma es colocando un apóstrofe y una **ese** ('s) al lado del propietario. Cuando el propietario es plural sólo se pone el apóstrofe.
e.g. John's book — el libro de Juan
The students' book — el libro de los estudiantes

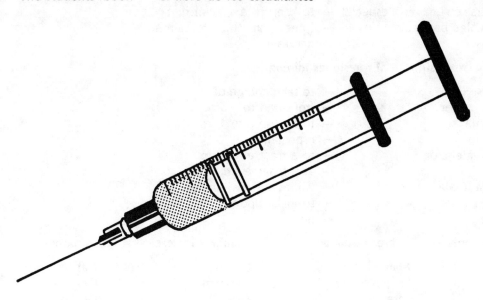

APPLIED VOCABULARY — VOCABULARIO APLICADO

The medicine has to be taken	**La medicina debe tomarse**
every hour	cada hora
every four hours	cada cuatro horas
according to what the doctor says	de acuerdo con lo que dice el doctor
according to the label	según la etiqueta
according to what the nurse says	según lo que dice la enfermera
according to your condition	según su condición
when needed	cuando la necesite
according to the prescription	según la receta
according to the symptoms	según los síntomas
according to how much pain you feel	según el dolor que sienta
according to your needs	según sus necesidades
1 tablespoonful	una cucharada
1/2 tablespoonful	media cucharada
1 teaspoonful	una cucharadita
1 pill	una pastilla

ADDITIONAL INFORMATION — INFORMACION ADICIONAL

1. Useful expressions — Expresiones útiles

Necesitar un especialista	— to need a specialist
Tener un dolor	— to feel a pain
Tener un fuerte resfriado	— to have a bad cold
Tener una enfermedad contagiosa	— to have a contagious disease
Favor de prepararme esta receta	— please make up this prescription for me
Mantenerse en una dieta especial	— to keep to a special diet
Necesito algo para calmar los nervios	— I need something to calm my nerves

2. Idiomatic expressions — Expresiones idiomáticas

Encargarse de	— to take charge of
De mal en peor	— from bad to worse
Dar lástima	— to arouse pity
Sobre todo	— especially
Llamar la atención	— to attract attention
A la vez	— at the same time
De buena (mala) gana	— willingly (unwillingly)
Insistir en	— to insist upon
Cerca de	— near

3. Spanish names — Nombres hispanos   Nombres ingleses — English names

Spanish names — Nombres hispanos		Nombres ingleses — English names	
Enrique	Manuela	Elaine	Gary
Germán	Santiago	Elizabeth	Gene
Juana	Sara	Ellen	George
Leonardo	Saúl	Emily	Gerald
Luz	Víctor	Erika	Glenn
		Esther	Gordon

4. Some sayings — Algunos refranes

Más vale tarde que nunca	— Better late than never
Más vale algo que nada	— Something's better than nothing
Poco a poco se va lejos	— Little by little one goes a long way
En boca cerrada no entran moscas	— Silence is golden
La práctica hace al maestro	— Practice makes perfect
El tiempo es oro	— Time is money
Amigo en la adversidad es amigo en verdad	— A friend in need is a friend indeed.
Más vale solo que mal acompañado	— It's better to travel alone than in bad company.
Antes que te cases mira lo que haces	— Marry in haste, repent at leisure.
Cuando una puerta se cierra otra se abre	— There's more than one way to skin a cat.
No dejes para mañana lo que puedes hacer hoy	— Don't put off until tomorrow what you can do today.
No hay rosas sin espinas	— Take the bitter with the sweet.
Quien busca halla	— He who seeks, finds.

5. Some common diseases — Algunas enfermedades comunes

absceso, postema	— abscess	epilepsia	— epilepsy
alcoholismo	— alcoholism	escaldadura	— diaper (or similarly caused) rash
amígdalas inflamadas	— swollen tonsils		
anemia	— anemia	escalofríos	— chills
apendicitis	— appendicitis	espinilla	— blackhead
apoplejía	— apoplexy, stroke	fiebre de heno	— hay fever
ataque al corazón	— heart attack	fiebre escarlatina	— sclarlet fever
bocio, coto	— goiter	fiebre reumática	— rheumatic fever
bronquitis	— bronchitis	gastroenteritis	— gastroenteritis
cáncer	— cancer	gonorrea, blenorragia	— gonorrhea
conjuntivitis	— conjunctivitis	granos, barros	— pimples
convulsión	— convulsion	hemorroides	— hemorrhoids
demencia	— insanity	hepatitis	— hepatitis
derrame de bilis	— gall bladder attack	herida	— wound
desangramiento, hemorragia	— bleeding, hemorrhage	hernia	— hernia
		histeria	— hysteria
desnutrición	— malnutrition	indigestión	— indigestion
desórdenes digestivos	— digestive disorders	influenza	— influenza
desórdenes respiratorios	— respiratory disorders	intoxicación	— intoxication
disentería	— dysentery	leucemia	— leukemia
distrofia muscular	— muscular dystrophy	llaga	— sore, fester
dolor de cuello	— stiff neck	malaria	— malaria
drogadicción	— drug addiction	meningitis	— meningitis
embolia cerebral	— cerebral ambolism	mononucleosis infecciosa	— mononucleosis
enfermedad coronaria aterosclerótica del corazón	— coronary atherosclerotic heart disease	menopausia	— menopause
		nauseas	— nausea
		neuritis ciática	— sciatic neuritis
enfermedades venéreas	— venereal diseases	peritonitis	— peritonitis
envenenamiento, intoxicación	— poisoning	piorrea	— pyorrhea
		polio o poliomielitis	— polio or poliomyelitis

prostatitis	— prostatitis	tuberculosis, tisis	— tuberculosis
pulmonía	— pneumonia	tuberculosis pulmonar	— pulmonary tuberculosis
retraso mental	— mental retardation		
reumatismo	— rheumatism	tumores	— tumors
sífilis	— syphilis	úlcera	— ulcer
sinusitis	— sinusitis	úlceras gástricas	— gastric ulcers
sordera	— deafness	urticaria	— urticaria, allergically caused itching welts on the skin
tétano	— tetanus		
tifus	— typhus		
tos	— cough	vaginitis	— vaginitis
tracoma	— trachoma	vómito	— vomiting
trombosis	— thrombosis		

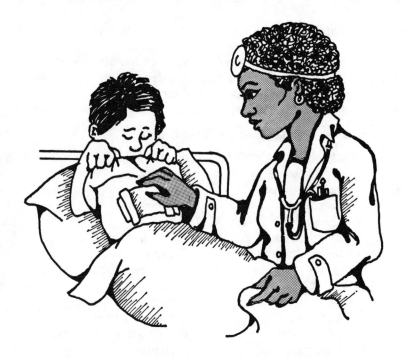

The Doctor and the Patient — El médico y el paciente

BILINGUAL PROJECT — PROYECTO BILINGUE

PREPARATORY EXERCISE 6 — EJERCICIO PREPARATORIO 6

The doctor asks the nurse to make a written report about the following case:

The patient's principal complaint is that of weakness, fatigue, and vague abdominal pain of several days' duration. He states that he has had some nausea but that there has been no vomiting, colic, or diarrhea. He has noted dark tarry stools over the past 3 days. He has felt some weakness and in spite of anorexia has been able to drink liquids and take some food.

El doctor le pide a la enfermera que haga un informe por escrito del caso siguiente:

Los síntomas principales del paciente son debilidad, fatiga y un dolor leve en el abdomen por varios días. Dice que ha tenido algunas náuseas, pero no ha tenido vómitos, cólicos ni diarrea. Dice que ha notado negro el excremento durante los tres últimos días. Se ha sentido un poco débil, y a pesar de la anorexia ha podido tomar líquidos y algo de comida.

```
┌──────────────────────────────────────────────────────────────────────┐
│                        REPORT __ INFORME                               │
│  NAME — NOMBRE ......................  HOSPITAL — HOSPITAL ...................  │
│  AGE — EDAD ..........................  ROOM No. — NUMERO DE CUARTO .........  │
│  SEX — SEXO ...........................  DATE — FECHA ........................  │
│  PHYSICIAN — MEDICO ..................  EXAMINATION —EXAMEN ...................  │
│  DIAGNOSIS — DIAGNOSTICO ...........  ......................................  │
│  ..........................................  ......................................  │
└──────────────────────────────────────────────────────────────────────┘
```

EXERCISES — EJERCICIOS

(Students learning Spanish — Estudiantes de español)

A. Rewrite the following sentences substituting the words on the right for the underlined words in the sentences. Make all necessary changes.

e.g. <u>Mi hermana</u> está enferma. Pedro y Juan están enfermos.   **Pedro y Juan**

1. <u>El paciente</u> dice mucho. ....   **yo**

2. <u>Yo</u> tengo un fuerte resfriado. ....   **tú**

3. <u>El laboratorista</u> es simpático. ....   **los técnicos**

4. <u>Ella</u> vive en la calle Colón. ....   **Luis y yo**

5. ¿Qué dice <u>la enfermera</u>? ....   **los policías**

B. Translate into Spanish.

1. Where is the nurse? ....   4. Where do you work? ....

2. I have a headache. ....   5. Today is Tuesday. ....

3. It's 2:30. ....   6. The nurse is intelligent. ....

C. Replace the English words with their Spanish equivalents.

e.g. Este es (**our**) apartamento.   <u>nuestro</u>

1. Francisco es (my) paciente.   _____

2. (Your, fam.) hermana es enfermera.   _____

3. Ellos tienen (their) recetas.   _____

4. ¿Conoce Ud. a (her) prima? Sí, señor, y también conozco a (his) hermano _____

5. Esta es mi medicina y esa es (yours, for.)   _____

D. Fill in the blanks by selecting the appropriate form in parenthesis.

e.g. Tienen <u>su</u> apartamento (**su, sus, suyos**).

1. Yo tengo _____ resultados médicos (mi, mis, el mío).

2. Este es mi diploma; ése es _____ (el suyo, los suyos, suyo).

3. Ella es una amiga _____ (nuestro, nuestros, nuestra).

4. El doctor atiende a _____ pacientes (sus, su, el suyo).

5. La anciana no _____ (oye, oigo, oyes).

EJERCICIOS — EXERCISES

(Estudiantes de inglés — Students learning English)

A. Traduzca las siguientes oraciones que indican propiedad.

1. El hospital de la ciudad. ....

2. La clínica del doctor. ....

3. Los pacientes del hospital. ....

4. La medicina de la enferma. ....

5. El libro del profesor. ....

B. Redacte seis oraciones con algunas de las expresiones idiomáticas que ya conoce.

1. ....   4. ....

2. ....   5. ....

3. ....   6. ....

C. Escriba un pequeño diálogo acerca de un paciente que consulta al doctor.

....

....

....

D. Llene los espacios vacíos con la forma apropiada del verbo en paréntesis.

1. The doctor _____ in the hospital. (work)

2. The nurse _____ a new uniform. (buy)

3. The patient _____ the bill. (pay)

4. I _____ a professional. (be)

5. He _____ five brothers. (have)

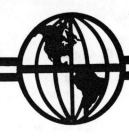

AT THE ADMISSIONS OFFICE
EN LA OFICINA DE ADMISIONES

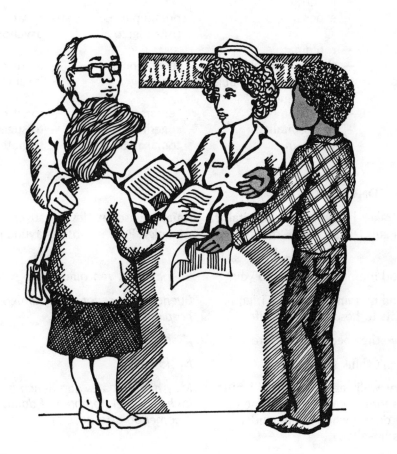

VOCABULARY — VOCABULARIO

A. Medical — Médico

admisiones	— admissions	llorar	— to cry
asegurar	— to insure	malestar	— discomfort
compañía de seguros	— insurance company	pagar	— to pay
cubrir	— to cover	planilla	— form
débil	— weak	póliza	— policy
delicado (a)	— medically serious	presión arterial elevada	— high blood pressure
deprimido	— depressed	prima	— insurance premium
doler	— to hurt	sano	— healthy
dormir	— to sleep	seguro social	— social security
los aseguradores	— the underwriters	sentir	— to feel
llenar	— to fill out	trastorno	— upset

B. General

atender	— to take care of	lugar	— place
avanzar	— to advance	poder	— to be able to, can
barato	— cheap	póliza nula	— invalid policy
camillero, asistente o ayudante médico	— orderly	preferir	— to prefer
caro	— expensive	preocuparse	— to worry
compañero de cuarto	— roommate	psicológico	— psychological
el consignatario	— the consignee	recomendar	— to recommend
el vencimiento	— the act of becoming or falling due	seguro	— insurance
excelente	— excellent	sentarse	— to sit down
hospitalizarse	— to hospitalize	sugerir	— to suggest
internar	— to intern	tomar nota	— to note down

CONVERSATION — CONVERSACION

A. Isaías Velásquez takes his wife to a hospital, and his friend Paul Jacobs, helps them by translating.

Isaías Velásquez lleva a su esposa al hospital, y su amigo Paul Jacobs les ayuda en la traducción.

Receptionist — Good morning, may I help you?

Buenos días, ¿en qué puedo servirles?

Paul — Good morning, miss, my friend wants to hospitalize his wife.

Buenos días, señorita, mi amigo quiere hospitalizar a su esposa.

Receptionist — Have they been here before?

¿Han estado aquí antes?

Paul — I don't think so.

No lo creo.

Receptionist — Very well, ask them to fill out this form including the name of the doctor who recommended this hospital.

Muy bien, pídales que llenen esta planilla incluyendo el nombre del doctor que les recomendó este hospital.

Paul — La señorita quiere que llenen ustedes esta planilla incluyendo el nombre del doctor que les recomendó el hospital.

The young lady wants you to fill out this form and include the name of the doctor who recommended this hospital.

Isaías — ¿Está en inglés o en español?

Is it in Spanish or English?

Paul — En inglés.

In English.

Isaías — Entonces vamos a llenarla juntos.

Then, let's fill it out together.

(They fill out the form.)

(Llenan la planilla).

Paul — Here it is all filled out.

Aquí está. Ya está llena.

Receptionist — Thank you. Would you please tell your friend he can take his wife to room 432. Everything is ready.

Gracias. Dígale por favor a su amigo que puede llevar a su esposa al cuarto núm. 432. Todo está listo.

Paul	— Puedes llevar a tu esposa al cuarto núm. 432. Todo está listo.	
Isaías	— Muchas gracias. Acompáñame.	*Thank you. Come with me.*
Paul	— Con gusto.	*With pleasure.*

GRAMMATICAL HINTS — APUNTES GRAMATICALES

A. There are some verbs in Spanish whose stem vowel changes. This occurs whenever the stem vowel is stressed. If the stressed vowel is an **e,** it changes to **ie** as in the verb **pensar:**

Yo p**ie**nso en español.   Nosotros pensamos en español.
Tú p**ie**nsas en español.
El
Ella p**ie**nsa en español.   Ellos
Ud.   Ellas p**ie**nsan en español.
                                  Uds.

These verbs are commonly referred to as **shoe** or **L** verbs because of the shape they take after the changed forms are grouped together. Some other verbs in this lesson with similar changes are: despertar, recomendar, querer, sentir, preferir, and requerir.

CONVERSATION — CONVERSACION (Cont.)

B. Fulgencio Reyes has medical insurance and the secretary asks him to sign the assignment of insurance benefits. His son Luis does the translation.

Fulgencio Reyes tiene seguro médico y la secretaria le pide que firme los papeles que autorizan los beneficios que recibirá. Su hijo Luis traduce.

Receptionist	— Sir, can you sign this authorization?	*Señor, ¿puede firmar esta autorización?*
Luis	— La señorita quiere que firmes esta autorización.	*The young lady wants you to sign this authorization.*
Fulgencio	— Con gusto, pero me gustaría saber de qué se trata.	*With pleasure, but I would like to know what it's about.*
Luis	— He wants to know what it's about.	
Receptionist	— This authorization says that the hospital can collect any payment related to the hospitalization of his wife, and if the insurance doesn't cover all expenses then he will be responsible for the remaining payment.	
Luis	— Esta autorización dice que el hospital puede cobrar cualquier pago relacionado con la hospitalización de tu esposa, y si el seguro no cubre todos los	

gastos entonces tú serás
responsable por el pago restante.

Fulgencio	— ¿Dónde hay qué firmar?	*Where shall I sign?*
Luis	— Aquí.	*Here.*
Receptionist	— Thank you.	
Fulgencio	— A sus órdenes.	*You are welcome.*

GRAMMATICAL HINTS — APUNTES GRAMATICALES (Cont.)

B. Sustantivos modificativos (noun adjuncts)

1. En inglés, al contrario de lo que sucede en español, un sustantivo puede calificar a otro sustantivo.
e.g. candy bar — una barra de dulce (nótese que en castellano se usa la preposición **de**).

C. En inglés se usa el sujeto **it** cuando uno se refiere a cosas, mientras que en español este sujeto está tácito.
e.g. It's a beautiful hospital — Es un hospital hermoso.
It's raining — Llueve.

D. Posición de los adjetivos (en inglés)

1. Por lo general los adjetivos preceden al sustantivo.
e.g. The brown hospital — El hospital café.
A large room — Un cuarto grande.

2. En preguntas, sin embargo, el sustantivo precede al adjetivo.
e.g. Is the clinic new? — ¿Es nueva la clínica?
Are the rooms small? — ¿Son pequeños los cuartos?

E. You have already learned in Section A that if the stressed vowel of a verb is an **e** it changes to **ie**. Another change is that when the stressed vowel is an **o** it changes to **ue** as in the verb **poder**.

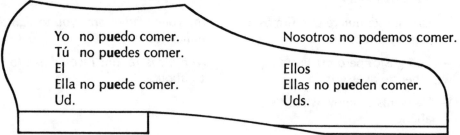

Yo no p**ue**do comer.   Nosotros no podemos comer.
Tú no p**ue**des comer.
El
Ella no p**ue**de comer.   Ellos
Ud.   Ellas no p**ue**den comer.
                                             Uds.

Again, if the changed forms are grouped, the result is a **shoe** shape or an **L** shape. Other verbs with such changes are: **dormir** and **morir**.

CONVERSATION — CONVERSACION (Cont.)

C. Dr. Harper asks Josefina Arroyo some questions; her husband Felipe does the translation.

El Dr. Harper le hace varias preguntas a Josefina Arroyo; su esposo Felipe se las traduce.

Dr. Harper	— How do you feel, Mrs. Arroyo?	*¿Cómo se siente, Sra. Arroyo?*
Felipe	— El doctor quiere saber cómo te sientes.	*The doctor wants to know how you feel.*

Josefina	—	Dile que anoche no dormí muy bien. Me duele el cuerpo. Me siento débil; y no puedo comer, aunque me muero de hambre.

Tell him that last night I didn't sleep to well. My body aches. I feel weak, and I can't eat, even though I am starving.

Felipe	—	She couldn't sleep last night. Her body aches. She feels weak and she can't eat even though she is starving to death.
Dr. Harper	—	I am going to examine you again.
Felipe	—	What do you think, doctor?
Dr. Harper	—	I don't think her case is very serious. It does require some attention. We'll take care of her illness.

No creo que su caso sea muy serio. Requiere, sí, algún poco de atención. Vamos a tratar su enfermedad.

Felipe	—	Dice el doctor que tu caso no es serio. Requiere apenas un poco de atención. El va a curar tu enfermedad.
Josefina	—	Dile que muchas gracias.

Tell him thanks.

Felipe	—	Thank you.
Dr. Harper	—	You're welcome.

GRAMMATICAL HINTS — APUNTES GRAMATICALES (Cont.)

F. Más contracciones

1. Como se ha observado en lecciones anteriores, en inglés se usan muchas contracciones. A continuación damos una lista de las más importantes.

are not	— aren't	do not	— don't	can not	— can't
is not	— isn't	does not	— doesn't	could not	— couldn't
was not	— wasn't	did not	— didn't	must not	— mustn't
were not	— weren't	will not	— won't	should not	— shouldn't

2. Otras contracciones usadas en oraciones positivas son:

I am	— I'm	I will	— I'll	I have	— I've
you are	— you're	you will	— you'll	you have	— you've
he is	— he's	etc.		etc.	
etc.					

e.g. I'm a student but I don't attend any school — soy estudiante pero no asisto a ninguna escuela.

G. Another change that often occurs in verbs is when the stressed vowel in the stem changes from an **e** to an **i** as in **pedir:**

Yo pido una planilla.   Nosotros pedimos una planilla.
Tú pides una planilla.
El
Ella pide una planilla.   Ellos
Ud.   Ellas piden una planilla.
                                             Uds.

Since the changes occur in the same forms of the verb as in the previous two groups, we can consider **pedir** a shoe verb also. Some other verbs that follow the same pattern are: rep**e**tir and s**e**rvir. The changes that occur in group A and in group E can take place in all three conjugations but this change (e > i) only happens in **-ir** verbs.

ADDITIONAL INFORMATION — INFORMACION ADICIONAL

1. Useful expressions — Expresiones útiles

Tenga la bondad de firmar aquí.	— Please sign here.	Me place oírlo	— I am pleased to hear it.
¿Cómo piensa pagar la cuenta?	— How do you intend to pay your bill?	Es muy bueno estar aquí.	— It's nice to be here.
¿Quién responde por usted?	— Who is responsible for you?	¿Cuál es su religión?	— What's your religion?
¿Cómo se llama su compañía de seguros?	— What's the name of your insurance company?	¿Cuál es el número de su seguro social?	— What's your Social Security number?
¿Quién es su agente?	— Who's your agent?	¿Dónde nació?	— Where were you born?
Lo siento mucho	— I am very sorry.	¿Quién le refirió?	— Who referred you?
Está bien	— That's all right.	Dar de alta	— Release from the hospital
Es usted muy amable	— You are very kind.		

2. Letter Writing — Escritura de cartas

Muy señor mío	— Dear sir	incluir, enviar adjunto	— to enclose
su atenta carta	— your letter	el mes pasado	— last month
en contestación a	— in answer to	presente, actual	— present
a vuelta de correo	— by return mail	que viene, entrante	— coming
sentir mucho	— to be very sorry	poner en conocimiento	— to inform
tan pronto como sea posible	— as soon as possible	en espera de contestación	— awaiting answer
por separado	— under separate cover	seguro servidor	— yours truly
		pormenores	— details
a sus órdenes	— at your service, you're welcome	a su debido tiempo	— in due time

3. Kinds of Insurances — Clases de seguros

contra incendios	— fire	de la triple A	— Triple A
contra robos	— theft	de plan de protección para la familia	— family plan
Cruz Azul	— Blue Cross		
de accidentes	— accident	de propiedad	— property
de ahorros	— savings	de responsabilidad civil	— liability
de automóvil	— car		
de cirujía	— surgical	de vida	— life
de choque	— collision	de viajes	— traveler's
de hipotecas	— mortgage	medicina general	— general medicine
de hospital	— hospital	personal	— individual
de incapacidad	— disability		

4. Spanish Names — Nombres hispánicos

Adolfo	Ernesto
Alfonso	Federico
Angélica	Hugo
Benjamín	Lidia
Dora	Mariela
Elvira	Ofelia

Nombres ingleses — English names

Gail	Jack
Gloria	Jane
Harold	Janet
Harry	Janice
Howard	Jeff
Isaac	Jenny

5. Idioms — Modismos

a pesar de, pese a	— in spite of
al mismo tiempo	— at the same time
al poco rato	— in a little while, shortly, a little later
bienvenido	— welcome
con cuidado	— with care

estrenar	— to wear, exhibit, etc., for the first time
hace tiempo que	— for a long time
por si acaso, por las dudas	— just in case
vaya con Dios	— May God be with you

6. More Vocabulary — Más vocabulario

despedirse	— to say goodbye
examen físico	— physical examination
guardar dinero, prendas o alhajas	— to put money, jewels, in a safe place

timbre	— bell, as a doorbell, an alarm bell
visita de médico	— doctor's visit

7. Bones of the Cranium — Huesos del cráneo

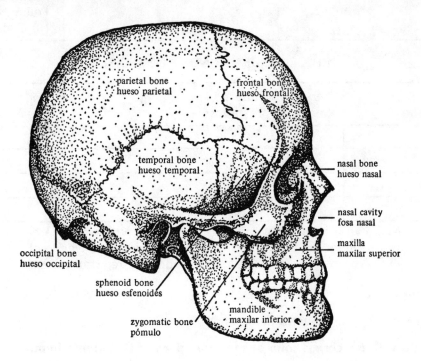

parietal bone
hueso parietal

frontal bone
hueso frontal

temporal bone
hueso temporal

nasal bone
hueso nasal

nasal cavity
fosa nasal

maxilla
maxilar superior

occipital bone
hueso occipital

sphenoid bone
hueso esfenoides

zygomatic bone
pómulo

mandible
maxilar inferior

BILINGUAL PROJECT — PROYECTO BILINGUE
PREPARATORY EXERCISE 7 — EJERCICIO PREPARATORIO 7

The registration form from the patient's first visit will become his first medical record.

El formulario de registro de la primera visita del paciente llegará a ser su primer registro médico.

REGISTRATION FORM PLANILLA DE INSCRIPCION			
Patient's Name — Nombre del paciente			Phone — Teléfono
Address — Dirección			
Date of Birth Fecha de nacimiento	Sex Sexo	Marital Status Estado civil	Social Sec. No. Núm. seguro soc.
Patient's Occupation Ocupación del paciente	Employer Patrón		Address Dirección
Name of Nearest Relative Nombre del familiar más cercano			Phone Tel.
Address of Above Dirección del mismo			
Insurance Co. Name Nombre Cía. de seguros			
Address Dirección			Policy No. Núm. de póliza
RECORD INDEX — INDICE DE REGISTRO			
Visit Date Fecha de visita	Services Rendered Servicios prestados		Code Clave

Make your own registration form, including the record index.

Haga su propia planilla de inscripción, incluyendo el índice de registro.

EXERCISES — EJERCICIOS

(Students learning Spanish — Estudiantes de español)

A. Fill in the blanks with the correct form of the verbs given in the infinite form.

1. El doctor (recomendar) _____ este hospital.

2. Ella (sentir) _____ miedo.

3. Nosotros (querer) _____ mejor sueldo.

4. Juan y Luis (negar) _____ la noticia.

5. Yo (empezar) _____ más tarde.

B. Fill in the blanks with the correct form of the verb given in the infinitive form.

1. La enferma (preferir) _____ estar en casa.

2. Los radiólogos (volver) _____ el martes.

3. El paciente (dormir) _____ profundamente.

4. Tú te (sentir) _____ mejor.

5. Uds. (mover) _____ los muebles.

C. Make a list in Spanish of all of the types of insurance you have.

. . . .

. . . .

. . . .

D. Answer in Spanish.

1. ¿Quién es su agente de seguros? . . . .

2. ¿Cuántas pólizas tiene usted? . . . .

3. ¿Qué piensa hacer usted durante las vacaciones de Navidad? . . . .

4. ¿Cuántas horas al día duerme usted? . . . .

5. ¿Cuál es el número de su seguro social? . . . .

E. Write a letter to an insurance company.

EJERCICIOS — EXERCISES

(Estudiantes de inglés — Students learning English).

A. Tradúzcanse las siguientes frases usando sustantivos modificativos.

1. Vendedor de medicina . . . .

2. Reloj de oro . . . .

3. Casa de madera . . . .

4. Caja de hierro . . . .

5. Edificio de cemento . . . .

B. Escriba cuatro oraciones en inglés usando el sujeto it.

1. . . . .   3. . . . .

2. . . . .   4. . . . .

C. Haga una lista en inglés de todos los planes o pólizas de seguros que tiene usted.

....

....

....

D. Traduzca estas oraciones al inglés.

1. ¿Viven los pacientes en la casa amarilla? ....

2. ¿Es un cuarto grande? ....

3. ¿Hay alumnos nuevos? ....

4. El libro rojo del profesor. ....

5. ¿Quién es el nuevo doctor del hospital? ....

E. Conteste las siguientes preguntas en inglés:

1. Who is your insurance agent? ....

2. How many insurance polices do you have? ....

3. What are you planning to do during Christmas vacation? ....

4. How many hours do you sleep? ....

5. What is your Social Security number? ....

F. Escriba una carta a alguna compañía de seguros.

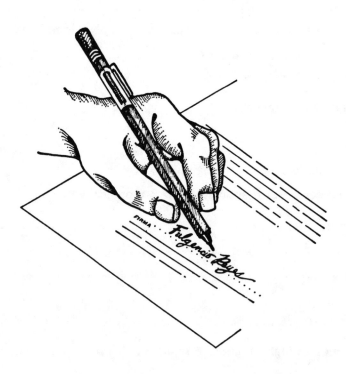

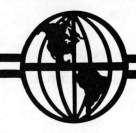

AT THE DRUGSTORE
EN LA FARMACIA

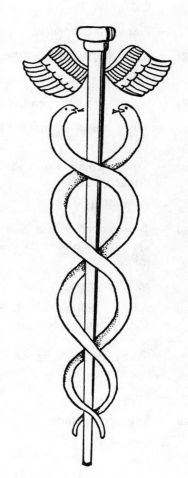

VOCABULARY — VOCABULARIO

A. Medical — Médico

alcohol	— alcohol
algodón	— cotton
amoníaco	— ammonia
aspirina	— aspirin
cloro	— bleach
desinfectante	— disinfectant
drogas	— drugs
farmacéutico	— pharmacist
farmacia, droguería, botica	— pharmacy, drugstore
gasa	— gauze
gotas	— drops
jabón	— soap
loción	— lotion
píldora, pastilla	— pill
quinina	— quinine
receta	— prescription
remedio, medicina	— medicine
ungüento	— ointment
vendaje	— bandage
yodo	— iodine

B. General

acordarse	— to remember
acostarse	— to go to bed
¿adónde?	— where?
afeitarse	— to shave
bañarse	— to take a bath
casero	— homemade
¿cuál?	— which?
gustos	— tastes, interests
invitar	— to invite
irse	— to go away
lavarse	— to wash oneself, wash up, get washed
levantarse	— to get up
oler	— to smell
peinarse	— to comb one's hair
pero	— but
solo	— alone
sólo, solamente	— only
trabajo	— work
vestirse	— to get dressed

CONVERSATION — CONVERSACION

A. Susana runs into Cristobal and Sandy on the street.

Susana se encuentra con Cristóbal y Sandy en la calle.

Cristóbal — Susana, ¿adónde vas tan a la carrera?

Susana, where are you going in such a hurry?

Susana — Cristóbal, voy a la farmacia y quiero llegar antes que cierren.

Cristobal, I am going to the drugstore, and I want to get there before they close.

Cristóbal — Susana, quisiera presentarte a mi amiga; ella vino de California.

Susana I would like to introduce you to my friend Sandy; she came from California.

Susana — Placer en conocerle.

Very happy to meet you.

Cristóbal — She is happy to meet you.

Está muy contenta de conocerte.

Sandy — I am happy to meet you too.

Cristóbal — ¿Qué vas a hacer en la farmacia?

¿What are you going to do in the drugstore?

Susana — Voy a buscar una receta para mi tía.

I am going to pick up a prescription for my aunt.

Cristóbal — Sandy, would you like to go to the drugstore also?

Sandy, ¿te gustaría ir también a la farmacia?

Sandy — I'd be delighted.

Me encantaría.

Cristóbal — Te acompañamos a la farmacia. Quiero comprar unos rollos para mi cámara.

We'll accompany you to the drugstore. I want to buy some rolls of film for my camera.

Susana — Muchas gracias.

Cristóbal — Además, allí hay una fuente de soda y pudiéramos tomar algún refresco.
Sandy, do you care for a cold drink?

Besides, there is a soda fountain there, and we could have something cold to drink.

Sandy, ¿quisieras tomar un refresco?

Sandy — Sure.

Claro que sí.

Cristóbal — Entonces, vamos.

Let's go then.

Susana — Vamos.

GRAMMATICAL HINTS — APUNTES GRAMATICALES

A. Present Participle and Progressive Construction

All verbs in the present participle form end in **-ndo.** The present participle of regular verbs is formed by taking the stem and adding **-ando** for the first conjugation and **-iendo** for the second and third conjugation.

comprar — comprando   comer — comiendo   vivir — viviendo

The present participle of irregular verbs is formed frequently in the same way. It is wise to remember that an unstressed **i** between two vowels becomes **y** and that the present participle will frequently end in **-yendo.**

  oír — oyendo creer — creyendo construir — construyendo

In the present participle of radical-changing verbs of the second and third class, the stem vowel changes from **o** to **u** or from **e** to **i.**

  morir — muriendo   mentir — mintiendo

To form the progressive construction, the present participle is used with the verb **estar,** signifying that an action is, was, or will be in progress.

  Estamos estudiando. We are studying.
  Están trabajando.   They are working.

Esta forma es también común en inglés: se usa muy a menudo y se forma añadiéndole **-ing** a la terminación del verbo. Cuando el verbo termina en una vocal, ésta se elimina.
  e.g. take — taking — tomando
    I am going to town tonight — Voy (estoy yendo) al pueblo esta noche.

CONVERSATION — CONVERSACION (Cont.)

B. Leonardo and Dick meet (run into, happen to meet) Javier at the bus stop and talk about their activities.

Leonardo y Dick se encuentran con Javier en la parada de los autobuses y hablan sobre sus actividades.

Leonardo — ¿Qué te pasa, Javier? ¿Porqué estás tan nervioso?

What's the matter, Javier? Why are you so nervous?

Javier — Es que si no viene el bus a tiempo voy a llegar tarde al trabajo. Entro a las ocho.

The fact is that if the bus doesn't arrive on time I'll be late to work. I start at eight.

Dick — It's already seven forty-five.

Ya son las siete y cuarenta y cinco.

Leonardo — It's getting late for him.

Ya se le está haciendo tarde.

Javier — I'm afraid so.

Así lo temo.

Leonardo — ¿A qué horas te levantas?

At what time do you get up?

Javier — Por lo general me levanto a las seis y media, pero hoy se me hizo tarde.

Usually I get up at six-thirty but I'm late today.

Dick — At what time do you get up, Leonardo.

Leonardo — Well, I get up at five-thirty, I read a while, I go jogging; when I get back I take a shower, shave, comb my hair, get dressed, and leave in plenty of time for work.

Bueno, yo me levanto a las cinco y media, leo un rato, salgo a correr; cuando regreso me baño, me rasuro, me peino, me visto y salgo para el trabajo con suficiente tiempo.

Dick — I follow more or less the same schedule, with the exception that I don't jog and I eat breakfast.

Yo sigo más o menos el mismo programa, con la excepción de que no corro, y tomo desayuno.

Leonardo	— I forgot to mention that I do eat breakfast.	*Se me olvidó mencionar que yo sí tomo desayuno.*
Javier	— Mi problema es que me acuesto bien tarde.	*My problem is that I go to bed quite late.*
Leonardo	— Mira, ahí viene tu autobús. Buena suerte.	*Look, there comes your bus. Good luck.*
Dick	— Good luck.	
Javier	— Gracias. Adiós.	

GRAMMATICAL HINTS — APUNTES GRAMATICALES (Cont.)

B. Reflexive verbs and pronouns

1. Basically a reflexive verb designates a verb whose subject and direct object are the same. In other words, the subject perfoms an action upon itself. This process is spelled out by the addition of reflexive pronouns to the verb.

$$\left.\begin{array}{l} \text{me levanto} \\ \text{te levantas} \\ \text{se levanta} \\ \text{nos levantamos} \\ \text{se levantan} \end{array}\right\} \quad \text{a las seis y media}$$

   Notice that the reflexive pronouns precede the verb.

2. Pronombres reflexivos en inglés.

   Los pronombres reflexivos son aquéllos que se refieren de nuevo al sujeto indicado. Estos pronombres son:

myself	e.g. I do it myself — Lo hago yo mismo.
yourself	
himself	John does it himself — Juan mismo lo hace.
herself	
itself	
ourselves	Mary cut herself on the hand.
yourselves	
themselves	The actor looked at himself in the mirror.

C. In Spanish the interrogative pronoun **cuál** means **which** (one) and normally asks for a certain one out of a number of similar things expressed or understood.

¿Cuál es tu hobby?
¿Cuál (de los deportes que se practican en la escuela) es tu deporte favorito?
¿Cuál es tu comida predilecta?

El pronombre interrogativo **which** puede referirse tanto a personas como a cosas, seleccionando a alguien o algo de entre un grupo determinado.
e.g. Which (of the books on the table) is your book? — ¿Cuál es tu libro?
     Which one is responsible for the trouble? — ¿Quién es responsable del problema?

CONVERSATION — CONVERSACION

C. Agapita, Olga, and Carmen talk about their hobbies.

Agapita, Olga y Carmen conversan acerca de sus aficiones, hobbies.

Olga	— ¿A dónde vas, Agapita?	*Where are you going, Agapita?*
Agapita	— Voy a la farmacia.	*I am going to the drugstore.*
Carmen	— ¿A comprar una medicina?	*To buy some medicine?*
Agapita	— No, voy a revelar unas fotos. Soy aficionada a la fotografía. ¿Cuál es la afición de ustedes?	*No, I am going to have some pictures developed; my hobby is photography. What's your hobby?*
Olga	— Tengo muchas: me gusta escribir cartas, leer libros, coleccionar estampillas, coleccionar tarjetas postales, viajar, arreglar flores y otras cosas más.	*I have many: I like to write letters, read books, collect stamps, collect post cards, travel, do flower arrangements, and some other things.*
Carmen	— Yo tengo sólo un hobby.	*I have only one hobby.*
Agapita	— ¿Cuál es?	*Which one is it?*
Carmen	— Me gusta aprender idiomas. Ahora estoy aprendiendo inglés.	*I like to learn languages. Now I am learning English.*
Agapita	— ¿Cómo se dice: "Tengo un dolor"?	*How do you say "I feel a pain"?*
Carmen	— I feel a pain.	
Olga	— ¿Cómo se dice "yo quiero ser enfermera"?	*How do you say, "I want to be a nurse"?*
Carmen	— Se dice: "I want to be a nurse".	
Agapita	— Muy bien. Esa es una lengua muy importante.	*Very good. That's a very important language.*
Olga	— Después nos vemos.	*See you later.*
Carmen	— See you later.	
Agapita	— See... you... later.	
Olga	— Adiós.	

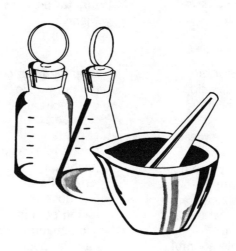

ADDITIONAL INFORMATION — INFORMACION ADICIONAL

1. Useful expressions — Expresiones útiles

¿Puedo cambiarle la venda? — Can I change your bandage?

¿Puedo limpiarle la herida? — Can I clean your wound?

Voy a cambiar la cama — I am going to change the sheets on the bed.

¿Hay una farmacia cerca? — Is there a pharmacy nearby?

Número de teléfono nocturno — night telephone number

Beba mucha agua — Drink plenty of water.

¿Le duele? — Does it hurt?

Consiga la medicina — Get the medicine.

¿Es adicto a las drogas? — Is he addicted to drugs?

¿Qué usa? — What do you use?

¿Qué síntomas tiene? — What symptoms do you have?

¿Tiene poco apetito? — Do you have a poor appetite?

Voy a ponerle una inyección — I'm going to give you an injection.

Tiene marcas de aguja — He has needle marks.

2. Some drugs — Algunas drogas

anfetaminas — amphetamines
aspirinas — aspirins
barbitúricos — barbiturates
cocaína — cocaine
codeína — codeine
demerol — demerol

LSD (ele ese de) — LSD
mariguana — marijuana
metadona — methadone
morfina — morphine
narcóticos — narcotics
penicilina — penicillin

3. Some other things found in a pharmacy — Otras cosas que se encuentran en la farmacia

cámaras fotográficas — cameras
cosméticos — cosmetics
crema dental — tooth paste
cuchillas para afeitar — razor blades
cheques de viajero — traveler's checks
dulces — candy
efectos de escritorio — stationery
espejuelos, anteojos — eye glasses
juguetes — toys

libros en rústica — paperback books
loción para broncear — suntan lotion
nueces — nuts
perfumes — perfumes
periódicos — newspapers
revistas — magazines
rollos de películas — rolls of films
tarjetas postales — post cards
tijeras — scissors

4. More vocabulary — Más vocabulario

aceite de castor — castor oil
ácido bórico — boric acid
al acostarse — at bedtime
alfiler — pin
antes de las comidas — before meals
antisépticos — antiseptics
cada dos horas — every two hours
cápsulas — capsules
con agua — with water
contra el consejo médico — against medical advice
cucharada — tablespoonful

después de las comidas — after meals
día por medio — every other day
dos veces al día — twice a day
esparadrapo — adhesive tape
etiqueta — label
imperdible, seguro — safety pin
jarabe para la tos — cough syrup
jeringuilla — syringe
líquido — liquid
loción para las quemaduras de sol — sunburn lotion
pastillas para la tos — cough drops

por la boca	— orally	tela adhesiva	— adhesive tape
solvente	— solvent	termómetro	— thermometer
tableta, pastilla	— tablet, pill	todos los días	— daily

5. Idioms — Modismos

aire, por favor	— let me have some air, please	hacer preguntas	— to ask questions
¡Cálmese!	— Calm yourself!	llevarse un chasco	— to be disappointed
faltarle a uno dinero	— to lack (need) money	manos a la obra	— let's get to work
		¡Oiga!	— Listen!
guardar cama	— to stay in bed	oír decir que	— to hear it said that
guardar silencio	— to keep silence (silent)	otra vez	— again
		salir el tiro por la culata	— to backfire

6. Spanish names — Nombres hispánicos

Algripina	Eduardo	Nombres Ingleses — English names	
Alicia	Isabel	Jennifer	Judy
Alonso	Jorge	Jill	Karen
Amparo	Josué	Jim	Keith
Clara	Ramón	Joan	Ken
Darío	Rosario	Jocelyn	Kenneth
Edgar	Teresa	Joe	Kent
		Julie	Kevin

7. More hobbies — Más aficiones, hobbies

| electrónica | — electronics | radioaficionado | — ham radio operator |
| escribir poesía | — write poetry | viajar | — to travel |

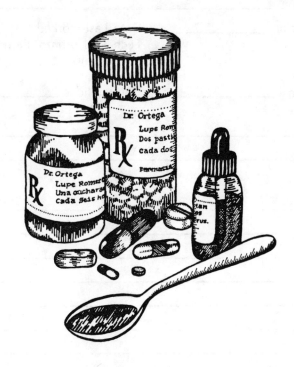

BILINGUAL PROJECT — PROYECTO BILINGUE

PREPARATORY EXERCISE 8 — EJERCICIO PREPARATORIO 8

Complete the medical data including chief complaints and present problems of the patient.

Complete el registro médico incluyendo el síntoma principal y los problemas actuales del paciente.

Hometown Hospital //09090

Alberto Lagler
562 Cochran Ave.
San Diego, CA 92154

Birthdate
Cumpleaños: 09—18—53

HOMETOWN HOSPITAL
  Hometown U.S.
  Medical Data Base
  History & Physical

Person Recording
Persona que registra: David López, M.D.
Time and Date
Tiempo y fecha: 12-30-80   10:30 p.m.

Age   Sex   Race   Marital Status
Edad_____   Sexo _____Raza_____   Estado Civil _____

Birth Place   Residence
Lugar de nacimiento _____   Domicilio _____

Education — Educación _____

Occupation — Ocupación _____   Date Last worked
                                          Fecha del último día en
                                          que trabajó_____

Source of information   Reliability
Fuente de información _____   Confiabilidad_____

Chief Complaint
Síntoma principal _____

_____

Present problems
Problemas actuales _____

_____

_____

_____

_____

_____

_____

EXERCISES — EJERCICIOS

(Students learning Spanish — Estudiantes de español)

A. Change the verb in each sentence to its progressive form.

1. Oigo la música. . . . .
2. Dormimos en el dormitorio. . . . .
3. Trabaja en la clínica. . . . .
4. Comen en la cafetería. . . . .
5. Compran las mercancías. . . . .

6. Muere el perro. . . . .
7. Estudiamos la lección. . . . .
8. Buscan al médico. . . . .
9. Escribes la carta. . . . .
10. Leo el libro. . . . .

B. Give the proper form of the infinitive given in parentheses.

1. Ella (levantarse) _____ temprano.
2. Nosotros (acostarse) _____ tarde.
3. Yo (acordarse) _____ de la tarea.
4. El paciente (lavarse) _____ las manos.
5. Tú (peinarse) _____ todos los días.

C. Make a list of things you can buy at the drugstore.

. . . .

. . . .

. . . .

D. Write six sentences using the interrogative cuál.

1. . . . .   4. . . . .

2. . . . .   5. . . . .

3. . . . .   6. . . . .

E. Translate into Spanish.

1. I have no hobbies. . . . .
2. I am going to the drugstore. . . . .
3. Which one is the patient you are talking about? . . . .
4. I need film for my camera. . . . .
5. Do you speak Portuguese? My friend does. . . . .

EJERCICIOS — EXERCISES

(Estudiantes de inglés — Students learning English)

A. Cambie las siguientes oraciones a la forma progresiva.

    1. I plan a trip. ....

    2. We sleep in the dormitory. ....

    3. The doctor works in the hospital. ....

    4. They eat at home. ....

    5. You swim in the swimming pool. ....

B. Haga una lista de las cosas que usted puede comprar en la farmacia.

    ....

    ....

    ....

C. Escriba seis oraciones usando which.

    1. ....   4. ....

    2. ....   5. ....

    3. ....   6. ....

D. Conteste las siguientes preguntas en inglés.

    1. What's your name? ....

    2. At what time do you get up? ....

    3. At what time do you go to work? ....

    4. What is your favorite dish? ....

    5. Which one is your brother? ....

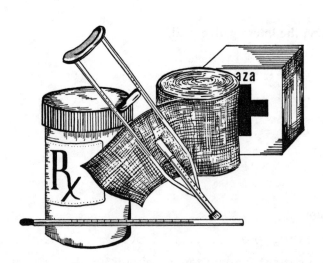

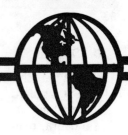

AT THE DENTIST'S OFFICE
EN EL CONSULTORIO DEL DENTISTA

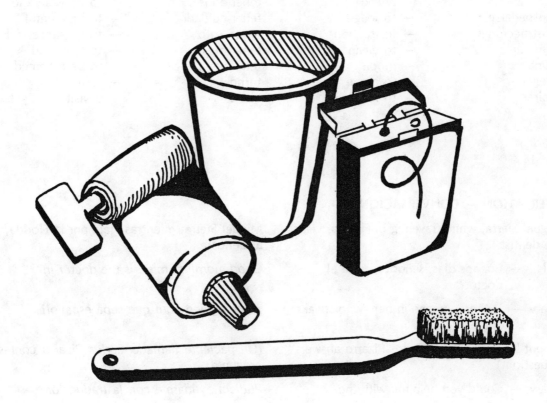

VOCABULARY — VOCABULARIO

A. Medical — Médico

absceso	— abscess	paladar	— palate
cepillo de dientes	— tooth brush	plata	— silver
consultorio del dentista	— dentist's office	pinzas	— tweezers
		porcelana	— porcelain
dentífrico, pasta de dientes	— dentifrice, tooth paste	puente	— bridge, bridgework
		radiografía	— radiography, X-ray photograph
dolor de muelas	— toothache		
emergencia	— emergency	raíz	— root
encía	— gum	rayos X	— X-rays
maxilar	— jaw	silla dental	— dental chair
oro	— gold	urgencia	— urgency

B. General

a la derecha	— to the (your) right	nitrógeno	— nitrogen
a la izquierda	— to the (your) left	por día	— per diem, per day
caminar	— to walk	rellenar, empastar,	— to fill (a tooth)
cuadra, manzana	— city block	emplomar, calzar	
derecho	— straight, straight ahead	tanto (a)	— so, as or so much
		tener años	— to be years old
hospedarse	— to lodge	tener cuidado	— to be careful
instrucciones	— instructions	tener éxito	— to be successful
limpiar	— to clean	tener miedo	— to be afraid
luna	— moon	tener vergüenza	— to be ashamed
llegar	— to arrive	turno	— turn
mirar	— to look	visita	— a visit

CONVERSATION — CONVERSACION

A. Miguel Sierra, while traveling in Florida, visits the dentist.

Miguel Sierra, mientras viaja por la Florida, visita al dentista.

Miguel — Buenos días, señorita, ¿está el doctor?

Good morning, miss, is the doctor in?

Secretary — Is there anyone in here who speaks Spanish?

¿Hay alguien aquí que sepa español?

(A patient by the name of Carlos Pizarro answers her question.)

(*Un paciente llamado Carlos Pizarro contesta la pregunta*).

Secretary — Could you help me with the translation?

Pudiera ayudarme con la traducción?

Carlos — With pleasure.

Con placer.

Secretary — Ask him what his problem is.

Pregúntele cuál es su problema.

Carlos — ¿Cuál es su problema?

Miguel — Dígale por favor que estoy de vacaciones, pero desde anoche tengo un fuerte dolor de muelas.

Please tell her I'm on vacation, but since last night I have had a very bad toothache.

Carlos — Since last night, he has been suffering a bad toothache.

Desde anoche padece un fuerte dolor de muelas.

Secretary — Please tell him he is very lucky because our office isn't full today. The doctor will see him soon.

Dígale por favor que tiene mucha suerte porque el consultorio no está lleno hoy. El doctor lo atenderá pronto.

Carlos — Tiene suerte. El doctor lo atenderá pronto.

You're lucky. The doctor will see you soon.

Miguel — Muchas gracias.

Carlos — De nada.

GRAMMATICAL HINTS — APUNTES GRAMATICALES

A. Tener

The basic meaning of **tener** is to have, to hold, to possess. However, this verb has other uses. It is used instead of the verb **to be** in expressions such as:

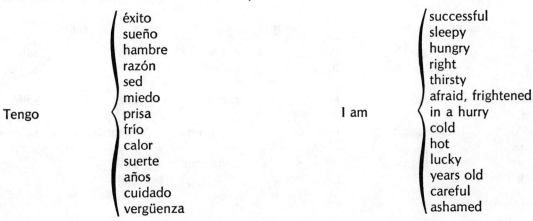

Tengo		I am	
	éxito		successful
	sueño		sleepy
	hambre		hungry
	razón		right
	sed		thirsty
	miedo		afraid, frightened
	prisa		in a hurry
	frío		cold
	calor		hot
	suerte		lucky
	años		years old
	cuidado		careful
	vergüenza		ashamed

The formula **tener que** + an infinitive is used to express obligation or necessity.

Ud. tiene que esperar — You have to wait
Tengo que trabajar — I have to (must) work

B. The preterite conjugation for **tener** is very irregular. It is as follows:

tuve   — I had
tuviste   — you (fam. sing.) had
tuvo   — he, she, you (for., sing.) had
tuvimos   — we had
tuvieron   — they, you (**fam., plu.**) had

C. El pretérito en inglés

1. El pretérito se usa cuando una acción comenzó en el pasado y terminó en el pasado.

2. El pretérito regular se forma añadiéndole **ed** a la terminación del verbo.
e.g. I work**ed** yesterday.

3. Se usa la misma forma con todas las personas del sujeto.
e.g. We worked yesterday.
He worked yesterday.

4. Si el verbo termina en una **e** se le añade sólo una **d.**
e.g. The surgeon operated on the patient.

5. El verbo **to be** es irregular en el pretérito.

I   was
you   were
he, she, it   was
we   were
they   were

6. El verbo **to be** se usa como auxiliar para expresar una idea continua en el pasado.
e.g. I was working at the hospital — Trabajaba en el hospital.

D. The preterite in Spanish

The preterite is a tense that expresses past actions or events which are seen as a whole, began in the past and were completed in the past. To form this tense, the infinitive ending (-**ar**, -**er**, -**ir**) is taken off and the special preterite endings are put in its place. In the case of the -**er** and -**ir** verbs, the endings are the same.

llegar		**comer**		**salir**	
yo	lleg**ué** *	yo	com**í**	yo	sal**í**
tú	lleg**aste**	tú	com**iste**	tú	sal**iste**
él		él		él	
ella	lleg**ó**	ella	com**ió**	ella	sal**ió**
Ud.		Ud.		Ud.	
nosotros	lleg**amos**	nosotros	com**imos**	nosotros	sal**imos**
ellos		ellos		ellos	
ellas	lleg**aron**	ellas	com**ieron**	ellas	sal**ieron**
Uds.		Uds.		Uds.	

CONVERSATION — CONVERSACION

B. Francisco Gutiérrez visits the dentist, Dr. Coleman. His secretary knows Spanish.

Francisco Gutiérrez viene a ver al dentista, Dr. Coleman. Su secretaria sabe español.

Francisco — Buenos días, señorita, ¿está el doctor?

Good morning, miss, is the doctor in?

Secretary — El doctor salió hace un momento, pero viene pronto. ¿Tiene usted una cita?

The doctor left a little while ago, but he is coming soon, do you have an appointment?

Francisco — No, señorita. Yo estaba de pasada y me detuve aquí porque tengo un fuerte dolor de muelas.

No, miss. I was just passing through and stopped here because I have a bad toothache.

Secretary — Aquí llega el doctor.

Here is the doctor.

Francisco — Qué bueno.

Good!

Secretary — This gentleman doesn't have an appointment, but he wants to see you because he has a bad toothache.

Este caballero no tiene una cita, pero quiere verlo porque tiene un fuerte dolor de muelas.

Dr. Coleman — Tell him to come in.

Dígale que pase.

Secretary — Dice el doctor que puede pasar.

The doctor says you can go in.

Francisco — Gracias.

Dr. Coleman —Tell me about your problem.

Dígame cuál es su problema.

Secretary — El doctor quiere saber cuál es su problema.

The doctor wants to know...

---

* In the form **llegué**, the **g** changes to **gu** before **e** to maintain the same hard **g** sound as in the infinitive llegar. Notice also the accent marks over the forms of the first and third persons singular.

Francisco — Resulta que ayer comí un helado con galletas y sentí dolor en una muela, y anoche no pude dormir muy bien.

What happened is that yesterday I ate ice cream and cookies and felt a pain in a back tooth, and last night I couldn't sleep too well.

Secretary — He has a toothache because he ate ice cream and cookies.

Dr. Coleman—Ask him to open his mouth.

Dígale que abra la boca.

Secretary — Abra la boca.

Dr. Coleman—We have to pull out that tooth.

Tenemos que sacarle esa muela.

Secretary — Le vamos a sacar la muela.

We are going to pull out the tooth.

Francisco — Está bien. Con tal de que se me quite el dolor.

That's fine; as long as the pain goes away.

A VISIT TO THE DENTIST — UNA VISITA AL DENTISTA

David Davis tells his friend Nancy about his visit to the dentist.

David Davis le cuenta a su amiga Nancy acerca de su visita al dentista.

Yesterday I went to the dentist's office, the one which is always full. I walked about four blocks before I got there. When it was my turn, the nurse pinned a protective napkin around my neck. She made me sit in the chair, started cleaning my teeth and took X-rays. When the doctor arrived, he looked at the X-rays and finished cleaning my teeth while giving me directions such as:

Ayer fui al consultorio del dentista, el cual está siempre lleno. Caminé unas cuatro cuadras hasta llegar allí. Cuando llegó mi turno la enfermera me puso un delantal al cuello para protegerme la camisa, me hizo sentar en la silla, empezó a limpiarme los dientes y me tomó unas radiografías. Cuando llegó el doctor, miró los rayos equis y terminó de limpiarme los dientes, mientras me daba algunas instrucciones tales como:

Open your mouth more	— abra más la boca.
Spit out, please	— escupa, por favor.
Please rinse your mouth out	— enjuágese la boca, por favor.
I am going to inject one side of your mouth to numb it.	— voy a ponerle una inyección para dormirle el lado.
Tap your teeth together	— golpee los dientes.
Move your head to this side	— mueva la cabeza para este lado.

ADDITIONAL INFORMATION — INFORMACION ADICIONAL

1. Useful Expressions — Expresiones útiles

¿Qué diente es el que le duele?	— Which tooth is it that hurts?	Quítese la dentadura (placa), por favor	— Please remove your dentures.
¿Le duele cuando mastica?	— Does it hurt when you chew?	Tenemos que sacarle la muela (el diente)	— We need to extract your tooth.
¿Le duele con lo frío y lo caliente?	— Is it sensitive to hot or cold?	Tenemos que rellenarle la muela (el diente)	— We need to fill your tooth.

¿Quisiera anestesia?	— Do you want an anesthetic?	Se le cayó la amalgama (el relleno)	— One of your fillings came out.
Cepíllese los dientes	— Brush your teeth.	Querer un relleno temporal	— To want a temporary filling
Cierre la boca un poco	— Close your mouth a little.	Los dientes postizos necesitan ser ajustados (reparados).	— The false teeth (denture) needs to be adjusted (repaired).
Tiene varias caries	— You have several cavities.		
Muerda fuerte	— Bite down hard.		
¿Tiene hambre?	— Are you hungry?	El puente se ha zafado	— The bridgework has broken loose.
¿Tiene sed?	— Are you thirsty?		
¿Tiene sueño?	— Are you sleepy?	¿Cree que puede arreglarse?	— Do you think it can be fixed?
Vamos a tomarle rayos equis	— We are going to take X-rays.	Un diente que debe sacarse	— A tooth that ought to be extracted.
¿Puede Ud. recomendar un buen dentista?	— Can you recommend a good dentist?	Un diente con absceso que debe ser curado	— An abscessed tooth to be treated.

2. More Vocabulary — Más vocabulario

amalgama	— amalgam	escupidera	— spittoon, cuspidor
anestesia local	— local anesthesia	espejo de dentista	— dental mirror
anestesia total	— total anesthesia	extracción	— extraction
caninos	— canine	frenillos	— dental braces
capilares	— capillaries	guardar cama	— to stay in bed, keep to one's bed
corona	— crown		
cuello del diente	— neck (of tooth)	incisivos	— front teeth
dentadura de adulto	— permanent teeth	inflamación	— inflammation
dentadura postiza, placas	— dentures, false teeth	molde	— mold
		muelas, molares	— molars
dentina	— dentine	nervio	— nerve
dientes de leche	— baby teeth	tenazas de extracción	— forceps
esmalte	— enamel		

3. Idioms — Modismos

a ambos lados	— on both sides	alguna cosa de actualidad	— current event
a buena hora	— in time, at the right time		
		algunas veces	— sometimes
a lo lejos	— in the distance	alguien me lo dijo	— someone told me
¿A quién le importa?	— Who cares?	alquilar un carro	— to rent a car
a tiempo	— on time, in time	echar a correr	— to start running
a toda velocidad	— at full speed	echar a llorar	— to start crying
abrir la puerta	— to open the door	echar a perder	— to spoil, ruin
abrir la ventana	— to open the window	no estar para la venta	— not for sale
agotado (a)	— exhausted	Ya es hora	— It is time.
al servicio de	— in the service of		

4. Idioms with the verb dar — Modismos con el verbo dar

dar de alta	— to dismiss from the hospital	dar la hora	— to strike the hour (said of clocks)
dar en algo	— to discover something	dar lástima	— to cause pity

dar que decir	— to make people talk or gossip	dar un abrazo	— to embrace, hug
dar que hacer	— to give a lot of trouble	dar un beso	— to kiss
dar risa	— to produce merriment, laughter	darse por muerto	— to consider oneself as good as dead
dar susto	— to frighten	darse por satisfecho	— to consider oneself satisfied

5. Spanish names — Nombres hispánicos   Nombres ingleses — English names

Abel	Marina	Kathy	Laurie
Carlota	Marcos	Kelly	Linda
Cecilia	Renata	Kimberly	Lisa
César	Rolando	Kirk	Loren
Edith	Soledad	Kurt	Lloyd
Javier	Vicente	Larry	Mark
Lucía	Yolanda	Laura	Marvin

6. Cross section of a tooth—Corte de un diente (sección)

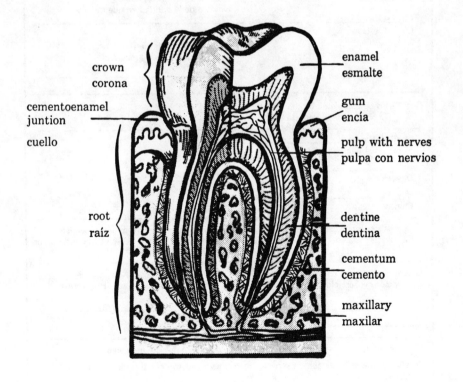

crown
corona

cementoenamel
juntion

cuello

root
raíz

enamel
esmalte

gum
encía

pulp with nerves
pulpa con nervios

dentine
dentina

cementum
cemento

maxillary
maxilar

BILINGUAL PROJECT — PROYECTO BILINGUE

PREPARATORY EXERCISE 9 — EJERCICIO PREPARATORIO 9

Below is a Dental Insurance Form. Fill out the complete form including the dental service rendered.

A continuación aparece un formulario de seguro dental. Llénelo incluyendo el servicio dental prestado.

NATIONAL INSURANCE COMPANY

Attending Dentist's Statement
Estado de cuenta del dentista que atendió

Insurance Co. use only
Sólo para uso de la compañía de seguros

Account No.   Pol/Plan
Cuenta núm.   Plan de póliza
_____   _____

Mail this form to:
Envie este formulario a:
                          National Insurance Co.
                          Box 943
                          Tacoma Park, MD 20012
Telephone (202) 723-0885
Teléfono

Part 1 – To be completed by Employee
Parte 1 – Debe llenarla el empleado

Name _____ Sex _____   Birthdate _____
Nombre   Sexo   Fecha de nacimiento

Address _____
Dirección   Employer (Company) name
                                      Nombre de la entidad en que trabaja
City, State _____
Ciudad, estado   _____

                                      Signature of the Insured
                                      Firma de la persona asegurada

                                      _____

Part 2 – To be completed by the dentist
        Debe llenarla el dentista

Dentist's Name _____
Nombre del dentista

Address _____
Dirección

City, State _____
Ciudad, Estado

Dentist's estimate _____   Dentist's statement of actual service
Cálculo del trabajo   Estado de cuenta del servicio prestado por
                                     el dentista

Description of Service   Date   Procedure No.   Fee
Descripción del Servicio   Fecha   Proceso núm.   Honorarios

_____   ____   ____   _____

_____   _____

I hereby certify that the procedures above were completed by date indicated.

Certifico por la presente que los servicios mencionados fueron completados en la fecha indicada.

_____ Date _____
         Signed (Dentist)   Fecha
         Firma del dentista

EXERCISES — EJERCICIOS

(Students learning Spanish — Estudiantes de español)

A. Translate the following into Spanish.

1. Are you cold? ....

2. I am 25 years old. ....

3. We are hungry and thirsty. ....

4. The dentist is right. ....

5. He is always wrong. ....

B. Fill in the blank with the proper form of the preterite according to the subject given (ar verbs).

1. Ayer la enfermera (visitar) _____ al niño enfermo.

2. En el comedor los laboratoristas (hablar) _____ de vacaciones.

3. Hace dos días yo (llevar) _____ a mi hijo al dentista.

4. Esta mañana mi primo y yo (comprar) _____ la receta.

5. El dentista (rellenar) _____ la muela.

C. Write six sentences using the verb tener in the preterite.

1. ....   4. ....

2. ....   5. ....

3. ....   6. ....

D. Answer in Spanish with complete sentences.

1. ¿Adónde va usted cuando tiene sueño? ....

2. ¿Qué hace usted cuando tiene hambre? ....

3. ¿Quién es su dentista? ....

4. ¿Cómo están sus dientes? ....

5. ¿Cuántas veces al día se cepilla usted los dientes? ....

E. Write a letter to your dentist making a complaint.

EJERCICIOS — EXERCISES

(Estudiantes de inglés — Students learning English)

A. Tradúzcanse al inglés las siguientes oraciones, prestando atención a los verbos en paréntesis.

1. Ella escuchó el programa. (listen to) ....

2. El técnico trabajó anoche. (work) ....

3. El doctor operó al paciente. (operate) ....

4. El atleta jugó al tenis. (play) ....

5. Yo practiqué la natación. (practice) ....

B. Formúlense seis preguntas en inglés.

1. ....   4. ....

2. ....   5. ....

3. ....   6. ....

C. Conteste a las siguientes preguntas en inglés.

1. What do you do when you have a toothache? ....

2. What is your dentist's name? ....

3. Do you have any cavities? ....

4. Why is gold so expensive? ....

5. How many teeth does a person have? ....

D. Escríbale una carta a su dentista protestando por la falta de buenos servicios.

E. Traduzca al inglés.

1. Tengo un dolor de muelas. ....

2. Necesito ir a ver a un dentista. ....

3. El dentista está muy ocupado. ....

4. El paciente le tiene miedo al dentista. ....

5. Estábamos escuchando el programa. ....

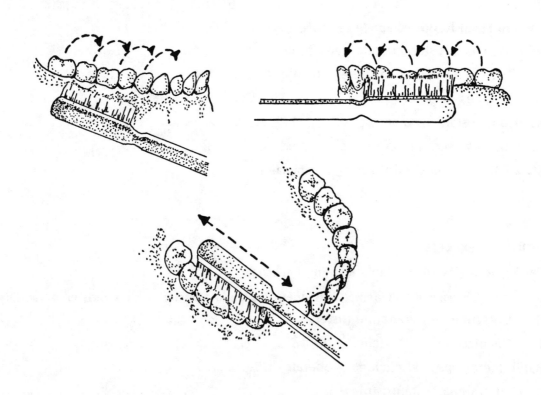

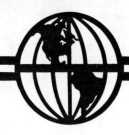

THE AMBULANCE
LA AMBULANCIA

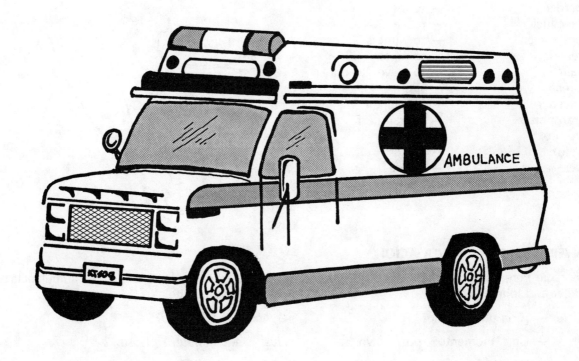

VOCABULARY — VOCABULARIO

A. Medical — Médico

anemia perniciosa	— pernicious anemia	manicomio	— insane asylum, madhouse
astillas en la piel	— splinters in the skin		
conducto lacrimal	— tear duct	pérdida de conocimiento	— loss of consciousness
coyunturas dolorosas, lastimadas	— aching joints	problemas familiares, personales	— family/personal problems
desarrollo tardío (del habla)	— delayed (speech) development	problemas financieros	— financial problems
desórdenes siquiátricos	— psychiatric disorders	pulmón de acero	— iron lung
dolor agudo	— sharp pain	sedante para dormir	— sedative for sleep
embolia cerebral	— cerebral embolism	silla de ruedas	— wheel chair
leucemia	— leukemia	tendón de Aquiles	— Achilles tendon
lunático	— lunatic	trombosis cerebral	— cerebral thrombosis
manía depresiva	— manic depressive	vómitos persistentes	— persistent vomiting

B. General

adolescente	— teen-ager	camioneta	— station wagon
atropellar	— to run over	cobrar	— to charge, collect

colonia	— district, colony
contrario (a)	— opposite
chocar	— to collide
enviar	— to send
escuchar	— to listen to
negocio	— business
perder	— to lose
precaución	— precaution
presenciar	— to witness
repetir	— to repeat
salir	— to leave, go out
sirena	— siren
suceder	— to happen
transportar	— to transport
vecino	— neighbor
veloz	— fast
ver	— to see

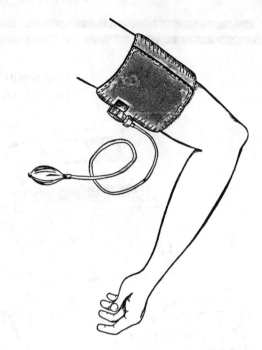

CONVERSATION — CONVERSACION

A. Horacio Perea calls the ambulance service of Peter and John White.

Horacio Perea llama al servicio de ambulancia de Peter y John White.

Horacio — ¿Con quién hablo?

Who am I talking to?

Peter — Un... momento... por... favor...

Just... a... minute... please...

John — What's the problem?

¿Cuál es el problema?

Peter — There is a man talking in Spanish.

Hay un señor que habla en español.

John — Let me see. After all, Spanish was my minor in college.
Hola... Bueno.

*Déjame ver. Después de todo el español fue mi menor en la universidad.
Hello...*

Horacio — Señor, ¿pudiera enviarnos una ambulancia a la Avenida Juárez núm. 32, en Colonia del Valle?

Mr., could you send us an ambulance to Juárez Avenue No. 32 in Colonia del Valle?

John — Repita la dirección, por favor.

Please repeat the address.

Horacio — Avenida Juárez, núm. 32.

John — Did you get the address, Peter?

¿Apuntaste la dirección, Peter?

Peter — Got it.

Ya la tengo.

John — ¿Cuál es el problema?

What is the problem?

Horacio — Tengo que llevar a mi esposa al hospital. Está para dar luz y ya le empezaron los dolores.

I have to take my wife to the hospital. She's about to have a baby and her pains have already begun.

John — Iremos en seguida.

We'll be right over.

Peter — Let's go.

Vámonos.

Traffic signs — Señales de tránsito

service and guide signs
señales informativas

CELAYA Cuota
S LUIS POTOSI →

REFORMA ↑ 57
95 ← INSURGENTES

E →

⛽ 1 km

🍴 500 m

✈ →

regulatory signs
señales restrictivas

ALTO

CEDA EL PASO

100 km/h MAXIMA

DOBLE CIRCULACION

industrial signs
señales industriales

PELIGRO
ALTO VOLTAJE

control boxes
controles

CONTROL DE SEMAFOROS

traffic lights
semáforos

warning signs
señales preventivas

GRAMMATICAL HINTS — APUNTES GRAMATICALES

A. Irregular preterites

1. In the previous lesson we mentioned that the preterite tense has special preterite endings which are attached to the stem of the infinitive. However, there are many verbs that have irregular stems and these verbs have a different set of endings.

poder			tener	
yo	pud**e**		yo	tuv**e**
tú	pud**iste**		tú	tuv**iste**
él ella Ud.	pud**o**		él ella Ud.	tuv**o**
nosotros	pud**imos**		nosotros	tuv**imos**
ellos ellas Uds.	pud**ieron**		ellos ellas Uds.	tuv**ieron**

2. Most of the irregular preterites usually have an irregular stem but the same set of endings, which vary from regular preterites only in two forms: first and third person singular. The strees is generally on the next to the last syllable, therefore are **no** written accents.

estar	(to be)	estuv-	-e	estuve
poner	(to put)	pus-	-iste	estuviste
querer	(to want to wish to love)	quis-	-o	estuvo estuvimos estuvieron
saber	(to know)	sup-	-imos	
venir	(to come)	vin-	-ieron	

3. The following three verbs have also one special irregularity each:

(decir)	dij-	dije	hice	traje
(hacer)	hic-	dijiste	hiciste	trajiste
(traer)	traj-	dijo	hi**zo**	trajo
		dijimos	hicimos	trajimos
		dij**eron**	hicieron	traj**eron**

4. Other special cases are the verbs **ir** and **ser** which are identical:

ir	ser
fui	fui
fuiste	fuiste
fue	fue
fuimos	fuimos
fueron	fueron

B. Most Commonly Used Irregular Verbs — Los verbos irregulares más comunes en inglés

Present	Past	Past Participle	Present	Past	Past Participle
arise	arose	arisen	forgive	forgave	forgiven
awake	awoke (awaked)	awoke (awaked or awoken)	freeze	froze	frozen
			get	got	gotten (got)
be	was	been	give	gave	given
bear	bore	borne (born)	go	went	gone
beat	beat	beaten	grow	grew	grown
become	became	become	hang	hung (hanged)	hung (hanged)
begin	began	begun	have	had	had
bend	bent	bent	hear	heard	heard
beseech	besought	besought	hide	hid	hidden (hid)
bid	bade (bid)	bid (bidden)	hit	hit	hit
bind	bound	bound	hold	held	held
bite	bit	bit (bitten)	hurt	hurt	hurt
bleed	bled	bled	keep	kept	kept
blow	blew	blown	kneel	knelt (kneeled)	knelt (kneeled)
break	broke	broken	knit	knit (knitted)	knit (knitted)
breed	bred	bred	know	knew	known
bring	brought	brought	lay	laid	laid
build	built	built	lead	led	led
burn	burnt (burned)	burnt (burned)	lean	leaned (leant)	leaned (leant)
burst	burst	burst	leap	leapt	leapt
buy	bought	bought	learn	learned (learnt)	learned (learnt)
cast	cast	cast	leave	left	left
catch	caught	caught	lend	lent	lent
choose	chose	chosen	lie	lay	lain
cling	clung	clung	light	lighted (lit)	lighted (lit)
come	came	come	lose	lost	lost
cost	cost	cost	make	made	made
creep	crept	crept	mean	meant	meant
cut	cut	cut	meet	met	met
deal	dealt	dealt	mistake	mistook	mistaken
dig	dug	dug	mow	mowed	mowed (mown)
do (he does)	did	done	pay	paid	paid
draw	drew	drawn	prove	proved	proved (proven)
dream	dreamt (dreamed)	dreamt (dreamed)	put	put	put
drink	drank	drunk	read	read	read
drive	drove	driven	rend	rent	rent
dwell	dwelt (dwelled)	dwelt (dwelled)	ride	rode	ridden
eat	ate	eaten	ring	rang	rung
fall	fell	fallen	rise	rose	risen
feed	fed	fed	run	ran	run
feel	felt	felt	saw	sawed	sawed (sawn)
fight	fought	fought	say	said	said
find	found	found	see	saw	seen
flee	fled	fled	seek	sought	sought
fling	flung	flung	sell	sold	sold
fly	flew	flown	send	sent	sent
forbid	forbade (forbad)	forbidden	set	set	set
forget	forgot	forgotten (forgot)	sew	sewed	sewn (sewed)

Present	Past	Past Participle	Present	Past	Past Participle
shake	shook	shaken	spring	sprang	sprung
shape	shaped	shaped	stand	stood	stood
shave	shaved	shaved (shaven)	steal	stole	stolen
shine	shone (shined)	shone (shined)	stick	stuck	stuck
shoot	shot ·	shot	sting	stung	stung
show	showed	shown (showed)	strew	strewed	strewed (strewn)
shred	shredded	shredded	strike	struck	struck
shrink	shrank	shrunk	string	strung	strung
shut	shut	shut	swear	swore	sworn
sing	sang	sung	sweat	sweated (sweat)	sweated (sweat)
sink	sank	sunk	sweep	swept	swept
sit	sat	sat	swell	swelled	swollen
sleep	slept	slept	swim	swam	swum
slide	slide	slid	take	took	taken
sling	slung	slung	teach	taught	taught
smell	smelled (smelt)	smelled (smelt)	tear	tore	torn
sow	sowed	sowed (sown)	tell	told	told
speak	spoke	spoken	think	thought	thought
speed	speeded (sped)	speeded (sped)	throw	threw	thrown
spell	spelled (spelt)	spelt	understand	understood	understood
spend	spent	spent	upset	upset	upset
spill	spilled (spilt)	spilled (spilt)	wear	wore	worn
spin	spun	spun	weave	wove	woven
spit	spit	spit	win	won	won
split	split	split	wind	wound	wound
spoil	spoiled (spoilt)	spoiled (spoilt)	withdraw	withdrew	withdrawn
spread	spread	spread	write	wrote	written

C. Cuando se hace una pregunta en el pasado se usa **did.**

    e.g. Did you go last night?

        ¿Fuiste anoche?

D. En oraciones negativas también se usa **did** —y las contracciones son muy comunes.

    e.g. I did not (didn't) go

        —No fui.

E. Adverbios — Adverbs

   1. La mayoría de los adverbios en inglés se forman añadiéndole **ly** al adjetivo.

      e.g. rapid   — rapidly   rápido   — rápidamente

           rigorous — rigorously   riguroso — rigurosamente

   2. Unas pocas palabras se pueden usar en ambas formas, ya sean adjetivos o adverbios. Estas palabras son: fast, slow, hard, late, early.

      e.g. She works hard — Ella trabaja duro.

           She is a hard worker — Ella es una trabajadora vigorosa.

   3. In Spanish you add **mente** to feminine adjectives to form adverbs.

      e.g. fácil, fácilmente — easily

           hermosa, hermosamente — beautifully

CONVERSATION — CONVERSACION

B. A policeman interviews Gary Johnson and his friend, Plácido García, who just came from Argentina.

Un policía entrevista a Gary Johnson y a su amigo Plácido García, quien acaba de llegar de la Argentina.

Policeman — Excuse me sir, did you see the accident?

Disculpe señor, ¿vió usted el accidente?

Gary — Yes, sir, I believe I witnessed everything.

Sí, señor, creo que lo presencié todo.

Policeman — In your opinion, how did it happen?

Según su opinión, ¿cómo ocurrió?

Gary — When my friend and I were coming out of my house, we heard a loud noise, and then we saw two cars, a station wagon and a sedan, crash in the middle of the intersection.

Cuando salíamos de mi casa oímos un fuerte ruido y entonces vimos dos carros, una vagoneta y un sedán chocar en plena bocacalle.

Policeman — Sir, when did the accident occur?

Señor, ¿cuándo ocurrió el accidente?

Gary — He doesn't know English.

El no sabe inglés.

Policeman — Ask him.

Pregúntele.

Gary — El señor agente quiere saber a qué hora ocurrió el accidente.

The policeman wants to know at what time the accident occurred.

Plácido — Yo diría que como a las seis de la mañana.

I would say about 6:00 a.m.

Policeman — Very well. I wonder if you would be willing to testify in court.

Muy bien, quisiera preguntarles si estarían dispuestos a declarar en la corte.

Gary — With pleasure.

Con gusto.

Policeman — Thank you.

ADDITIONAL INFORMATION — INFORMACION ADICIONAL

1. Some parts of a car — Algunas piezas del automóvil

acelerador	— accelerator	chispa	— spark
aceite	— oil	eje	— axle
aire acondicionado	— air-conditioned, air conditioning	faros	— headlights
bocina, pito	— horn	freno	— brake
bomba de aire	— air pump	luces	— lights
bujía	— spark plug	llanta, goma	— tire
caja de velocidades	— gear box	motor	— engine
carburador	— carburetor	radiador	— radiator
cigüeñal	— crankshaft	resorte	— spring
cojinete, rodamiento de bolas	— ball bearing	tanque	— tank
		válvula	— valve
chasís	— car frame, chassis	volante, timón	— steering wheel

2. Some professions — Algunas profesiones

abogado	— lawyer	maestro, profesor	— teacher
agricultor	— farmer	mecánico	— mechanic
albañil	— bricklayer	ministro	— minister
arquitecto	— architect	modista	— dressmaker
aviador, piloto	— aviator, pilot	pintor	— painter
carnicero	— butcher	panadero	— baker
carpintero	— carpenter	plomero, fontanero	— plumber
cocinero	— cook	relojero	— watchmaker, watch repairman
comerciante	— businessman		
chofer	— chauffeur, driver	sastre	— tailor
escritor	— writer	trabajador social	— social worker
fotógrafo	— photographer	zapatero	— shoemaker, shoe repairman
impresor	— printer		
locutor	— announcer		

3. Useful expressions — Expresiones útiles

¿Qué clase de automóvil tiene Ud.?	— What kind of car do you have?
¿Cuáles son las leyes de tránsito?	— What are the traffic regulations?
Llame una ambulancia, por favor	— Please call an ambulance.
¿Conoce Ud. a un buen mecánico?	— Do you know a good mechanic?
¿Qué clase de gasolina usa?	— What kind of gasoline does it take?
¿Cuántos caballos de fuerza?	— How many horse power?
¿Conoce Ud. el camino?	— Do you know the road (way)?
Llévenos a…	— Drive us to…
Indíqueme, por favor, qué camino seguir.	— Please show me what road to follow.
¿Cuántas horas tomará en ir y venir?	— How many hours will it take to get there and back?
¿Es un buen camino?	— Is it a good road?
¿Puedo estacionarme aquí?	— May I park here?
¿Hay un buen garaje por aquí cerca?	— Is there a good garage nearby?
¿Puede Ud. dirigirnos al hospital?	— Can you direct us to the hospital?

4. Idioms — Modismos

Cálmese	— Calm yourself. Calm down.	dar un paseo	— to go for a ride, a walk
cambiar dinero	— to change or exchange money	de allí en adelante	— thereafter
		de aquí en adelante	— hereafter
cambiarse de ropa	— to change clothes	de carne y hueso	— real, of flesh and blood
como de costumbre	— as usual		
¿Cómo se siente hoy?	— How do you feel today?	de veras	— really, truly
		de vez en cuando	— once in a while
con su permiso	— with your permission	de visita	— making a call
		directorio telefónico	— telephone directory, telephone book
¡Cuánto lo siento!	— I am so sorry!		
dar la vuelta	— to go around	guía telefónica	— telephone directory, telephone book

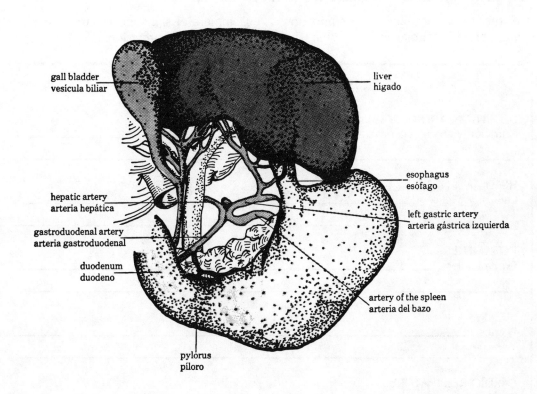

gall bladder
vesícula biliar

liver
hígado

esophagus
esófago

hepatic artery
arteria hepática

left gastric artery
arteria gástrica izquierda

gastroduodenal artery
arteria gastroduodenal

duodenum
duodeno

artery of the spleen
arteria del bazo

pylorus
píloro

5. Spanish names — Nombres hispanos

Alba	Leopoldo
Amanda	Mauricio
Augusto	Miguel
Emilio	Nicandro
Estela	Piedad
Graciela	Tomás
Guillermo	Yolanda

Nombres ingleses — English names

Lois	Niel
Margaret	Nick
Melody	Norman
Melvin	Pam
Michael	Pamela
Mike	Patricia
Monty	Patty

6. More vocabulary — Más vocabulario

batería	— battery	lavar	— to wash
calentador, calentón	— heater	licencia para manejar	— driver's license
dar brillo	— to polish	número de la placa	— Licence plate or tag number
en la estación de policía	— At the police station		
encerar	— to wax	poner en marcha, arrancar (el motor)	— to start (a car or a motor)
engrasar	— to grease	reparar	— to repair

BILINGUAL PROJECT — PROYECTO BILINGUE

PREPARATORY EXERCISE 10 — EJERCICIO PREPARATORIO 10

Complete the following physical examination, including the provisional diagnosis.

Complete el siguiente examen físico incluyendo el diagnóstico provisional.

PHYSICAL EXAMINATION
EXAMEN FISICO

NUTRITION AND GENERAL APPEARANCE
Nutrición y apariencia general _____

_____

HEAD AND NECK
Cabeza y cuello _____

_____

EXTREMITIES
Extremidades _____

_____

BREASTS
Pechos _____

_____

CARDIO-RESPIRATORY
Cardiorespiratorio _____

_____

GASTROINTESTINAL _____

_____

NEUROMUSCULAR _____

_____

BONES, JOINTS, AND SKIN
Huesos, coyunturas y piel _____

_____

GLANDS
Glándulas _____

_____

PROVISIONAL DIAGNOSIS
Diagnóstico Provisional _____

_____

Signed: _____ MD _____
Firma:

EXERCISES — EJERCICIOS

(Students learning Spanish — Estudiantes de español)

A. Give the proper preterite form of the verbs in parentheses.

1. Ella (tener) _____ un fuerte dolor de garganta.

2. Los enfermos (ir) _____ a la casa.

3. El doctor (poder) _____ hacer la operación.

4. Los laboratoristas no (trabajar) _____ ayer.

5. Yo (salir) _____ temprano ayer.

B. Translate into Spanish.

1. They came early to school. . . . .

2. The supervisor did not want to see the accident. . . . .

3. What did you say? . . . .

4. I didn't know that. . . . .

5. The orderly brought the patient. . . . .

C. Write a dialogue concerning your visit to a mechanic in which you explain your car's problem.

. . . .

. . . .

. . . .

D. Make a list in Spanish of some of your relatives and their professions.

. . . .

. . . .

. . . .

E. Write six sentences in Spanish using irregular verbs in the preterite.

1. . . . .   4. . . . .

2. . . . .   5. . . . .

3. . . . .   6. . . . .

F. Answer in Spanish in complete sentences.

1. ¿Qué clase de automóvil tiene usted? . . . .

2. ¿Cómo es el motor de su vehículo? . . . .

3. ¿Cuál es el número de teléfono de la ambulancia? . . . .

4. ¿Quién se quebró un brazo en su familia? . . . .

5. ¿Cuándo fué la última vez que tomó usted un examen físico? . . . .

EJERCICIOS — EXERCISES
(Estudiantes de inglés — Students learning English)

A. Escriba seis oraciones usando verbos irregulares en el pretérito.

   1. ....   4. ....

   2. ....   5. ....

   3. ....   6. ....

B. Busque seis adjetivos, transfórmelos luego en adverbios y después haga oraciones con ellos.

   1. ....   4. ....

   2. ....   5. ....

   3. ....   6. ....

C. Escriba un diálogo concerniente a una visita al mecánico en el que le explique los problemas que tiene su carro.

D. Conteste las siguientes preguntas en inglés.

   1. Did you buy the medicine for the patient? ....

   2. What kind of car do you have? ....

   3. Who was involved in the accident? ....

   4. Did you sleep well last night? ....

   5. Where did you eat yesterday? ....

E. Llene los espacios vacíos con el pretérito de los verbos dados entre paréntesis.

   1. Mr. Johnston _____ (leave) for Mexico yesterday.

   2. The patients _____ (come) to the clinic a month ago.

   3. The doctor _____ (arrive) on time.

   4. The boy _____ (cuts) his finger.

   5. We _____ (meet) last night.

F. Traduzca al inglés.

   1. Mi carro tiene un motor grande. ....

   2. Anoche tuvimos que llamar a la ambulancia. ....

   3. Me quebré un brazo esquiando en la nieve. ....

   4. Anoche salimos temprano. ....

   5. El fue al concierto con mi hermana. ....

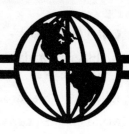

EMERGENCIES: FIRST-AID
EMERGENCIAS: PRIMEROS AUXILIOS

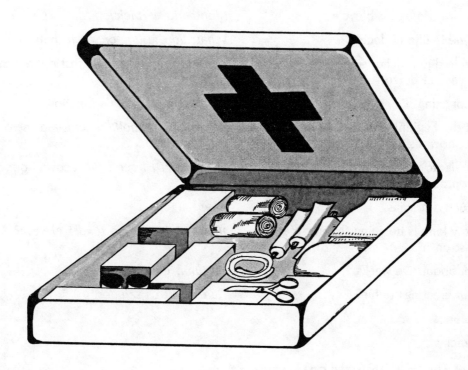

VOCABULARY — VOCABULARIO

A. Medical — Médico

acidosis	— acidosis	pulso	— pulse
ahogarse	— to drown	quemaduras	— burns
camilla	— stretcher	respiración artificial	— artificial respiration
está sangrando	— He (she) is bleeding	sala de emergencias	— emergency room
estado de coma	— in a coma	salvavidas	— life guard, life preserver
enyesar	— to put on, apply a plaster cast	temblores	— tremors
fatiga	— fatigue		

B. General

andamio	— scaffold	isla	— island
botón	— button	ladrón	— thief
buscar	— to look for	llamar	— to call
caer, caerse	— to fall, fall down	moneda	— coin
etiqueta	— label	obrero	— workman
frasco	— bottle	recoger	— to pick up
inconsciente	— unconscious	respirar	— to breathe
infeliz	— unhappy, poor soul	torero	— bullfighter

CONVERSATION — CONVERSACION

A. Juliana, María and Thelma talk at the university.

Juliana, María y Thelma conversan cerca de la universidad.

Juliana — María, ¿qué le pasó a tu hermanito?	*María, what happened to your little brother?*
María — Se cayó y se rompió un brazo.	*He fell and broke an (his) arm.*
Thelma — What was he doing?	*¿Qué estaba haciendo?*
María — He was riding his bicycle.	*Montando en bicicleta.*
Juliana — ¿Qué le dijo el doctor?	*What did the doctor say to him?*
María — No le dijo mucho; solamente le enyesó el brazo.	*He didn't say much. He just put a cast on it.*
Thelma — Poor thing! Does it hurt much?	*¡Pobrecito! ¿Le duele mucho?*
María — At the beginning it hurt very much, but now it's not too (so) bad.	*Al principio le dolía muchísimo, pero ahora no está tan malo.*
Juliana — Lo siento mucho. Que se mejore pronto.	*I am sorry. I hope he'll recover soon.*
María — Muchas gracias.	
Thelma — How long is he going to have the cast on it?	*¿Por cuánto tiempo tendrá el yeso?*
María — For about five weeks.	*Por unas cinco semanas.*
Thelma — Our greetings to him.	*Dale nuestros saludos.*
Juliana — Saludos.	
María — Gracias.	

GRAMMATICAL HINTS — APUNTES GRAMATICALES

A. The preterite form of the verb **caer** and other verbs of this kind goes like this:

caí	— I fell
caíste	— you (fam. sing.) fell
cayó	— he, she, it, you (for. sing.) fell
caímos	— we fell
cayeron	— they, you (plu.) fell

B. Acabar de plus an infinitive means **to have just** plus a past participle.
e.g. Acabo de llegar — I just came (I have just come.)
Acabamos de recibir una carta — we just received a letter.

C. Adjetivos y pronombres demostrativos

1. This y **that** son palabras demostrativas porque señalan algo.
This (este, esta) se usa para referirse a una cosa que está cerca de la persona que habla; **that** se usa para referirse a una cosa que está lejos de la persona que habla, y significa: ese, esa, aquel, aquella.
e.g. This book is mine — este libro es mío.
that book is yours — ese libro es tuyo.

2. El plural de estos demostrativos es **these** (estos, estas) y **those** (esos, esas, aquellos, aquellas).
e.g. these medicines — estas medicinas.

3. Cuando se reemplaza el sustantivo por un pronombre entonces se le añade **one** o **ones.**
e.g. This book is mine; that **one** is yours.

D. Demonstrative adjectives and pronouns

The demonstrative adjectives point out persons or objects. Every time a demonstrative adjective is used to modify a noun, it is repeated before the noun. Demonstrative adjectives vary according to the number and gender of the nouns that they modify. They also vary according to the distance in space, time, and even thought between the speaker and the persons or objects.

Este and **esta** mean near the person speaking; **ese** and **esa** mean distant-frequently near the person spoken to; and **aquel** and **aquella** mean farther away-distant from both speaker and person spoken to.

este	lápiz	(this)	**esta**	pluma	(near)
ese	lápiz	(that)	**esa**	pluma	(far away)
aquel	lápiz	(that)	**aquella**	pluma	(farther away)
estos	lápices	(these)	**estas**	plumas	(near)
esos	lápices	(those)	**esas**	plumas	(far away)
aquellos	lápices	(those)	**aquellas**	plumas	(farther away)

Demonstrative pronouns are the same as demonstrative adjectives except for a difference in the written form. They are distinguished by the accent they bear, although it may be left off if the context is clear.

este libro	**éste**	esta silla	**ésta**
ese libro	**ése**	esa silla	**ésa**
aquel libro	**aquél**	aquella silla	**aquélla**
estos libros	**éstos**	estas sillas	**éstas**
esos libros	**ésos**	esas sillas	**ésas**
aquellos libros	**aquéllos**	aquellas sillas	**aquéllas**

Neuter demonstrative pronouns do not need an accent, because they do not have corresponding adjective forms.

esto   **eso**   **aquello**

e.g. ¿Qué es eso? — What's that?

E. Más preposiciones — More prepositions

from (de) Indica procedencia. e.g. Where are you **from**? — ¿De dónde es Ud.?

with (con) e.g. He is coming **with** me — Viene conmigo.

about (acerca de) e.g. She likes to talk **about** her work — A ella le gusta hablar acerca de su trabajo.

in (en) e.g. The doctor lives **in** a large city — El médico vive en una ciudad grande.

at (en el, en la, en los, en las, etc.) Localiza y sitúa con precisión.
e.g. John and Peter are roommates **at** the university —
Juan y Pedro son compañeros de cuarto **en** la universidad.

to (a) Esta preposición se usa con verbos de movimiento y con otros verbos. Indica también el complemento indirecto.
e.g. Bill goes **to** the hospital — Bill va al hospital.
Bruce is introducing Tom **to** his family — Bruce presenta Tom a su familia.
Joe gives the book **to** his father — Joe le da el libro a su padre (complemento indirecto).

CONVERSATION — CONVERSACION (Cont.)

B. Berta and little June, her sister, are swimming in a lake, and Berta meets her friend Alice, who is learning Spanish.

Berta y su hermanita June están nadando en un lago, y Berta se encuentra con su amiga Alice, que está aprendiendo español.

Alice — I wonder what is going on over there.

Me pregunto qué estará pasando allá.

Berta — I don't know... pero hablemos en español.

No sé... but let's speak in Spanish.

Alice — Allá está el salvavidas...

There is the lifeguard.

Berta — I wonder if someone is drowning.

Me pregunto si alguien se está ahogando.

Alice — I don't know... What about speaking in Spanish?

No sé... ¿No vamos a hablar en español?

Berta — Perdona... estoy un poco preocupada... ¿dónde está mi hermanita June?

I'm sorry... I am a little worried... where is my sister June?

Alice — No sé... la última vez que la vi estaba nadando allá donde está la gente.

I don't know... the last time I saw her she was swimming over there where the people are.

Berta — You don't say... She is the one drowning.

No me digas... Ella es la que se está ahogando.

(Meanwhile the lifeguard has brought June to shore.)

(Mientras tanto el salvavidas ha traído a June a la orilla.)

Berta — Señor, ¿cree usted que vivirá?

Do you think she'll live?

Salvavidas — Creo que sí... su amiga le está dando respiración artificial.

I think so... your friend is giving her artificial respiration.

Berta — How is my sister, Alice?

¿Cómo está mi hermana, Alice?

Alice — She is getting back to normal now.

Ya se está normalizando.

Salvavidas — I think she is all right.

Creo que ya está bien.

Berta — ¡Qué susto! Por un momento pensé que se moriría.

How frightening! For a moment I thought she would die.

Salvavidas — Ya está mejor, pero mantenga la vista en ella por un rato.

She is better, but keep an eye on her for a while.

Berta — Muchas gracias, señor. Let's go Alice.

Thank you, sir. Vámonos Alice.

GRAMMATICAL HINTS — APUNTES GRAMATICALES (Cont.)

F. Otros verbos ingleses — Other English Verbs

Algunos verbos, tales como **prefer** (preferir), **want** (querer), **like** (gustar), **need** (necesitar) y **begin** (comenzar) se forman poniéndoles **to** después de la forma verbal o inmediatamente antes del infinitivo.

e.g. The sick man wants to go outdoors — el enfermo quiere salir.

What do you need to buy? — ¿Qué quieres comprar?

AN ACCIDENT — UN ACCIDENTE

Flora Duncan tells her friend Mary about an accident.

Dr. Felix Day had just arrived at the hospital. He was called on emergency because there had occurred a terrible accident. A worker fell from a scaffold and was plunged into a state of prolonged unconsciousness. He seemed to have several broken ribs, and perhaps internal injuries, because he was expelling blood orally. The nurse laid him on a table, and as soon as the doctor entered, the poor fellow, who was regaining consciousness, began to complain pitifully. When the doctor arrived the ambulance was leaving.

Flora Duncan le cuenta a su amiga Mary acerca de un accidente.

El doctor Felix Day acaba de llegar al hospital. Lo llamaron porque acababa de suceder un terrible accidente, y tuvo que venir de emergencia. Un obrero se cayó de un andamio y quedó inconsciente, en estado de coma. Parece que se le rompieron varias costillas, tal vez tenga lesiones internas porque echa sangre por la boca. La enfermera lo acostó en una mesa y cuando llegó el doctor, el infeliz, que ya estaba volviendo en sí, se quejaba profundamente. Cuando el doctor llegó, la ambulancia ya salía de nuevo.

The Skeleton — El esqueleto

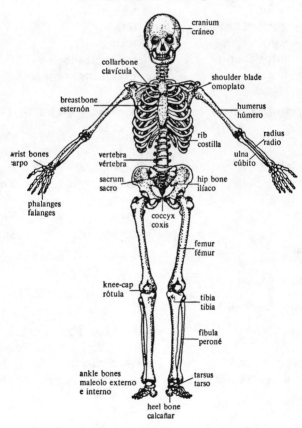

cranium
cráneo

collarbone
clavícula

shoulder blade
omoplato

breastbone
esternón

humerus
húmero

rib
costilla

radius
radio

wrist bones
carpo

vertebra
vértebra

ulna
cúbito

sacrum
sacro

hip bone
ilíaco

phalanges
falanges

coccyx
coxis

femur
fémur

knee-cap
rótula

tibia
tibia

fibula
peroné

ankle bones
maleolo externo
e interno

tarsus
tarso

heel bone
calcañar

ADDITIONAL INFORMATION — INFORMACION ADICIONAL

1. Emergencies, Accidents — Emergencias, accidentes

ataque	— attack	mala caída	— a bad fall
aturdimiento	— bewilderment, dizziness	mordedura de perro	— dog bite
caída	— fall	mordedura de serpiente	— snake bite
calambre	— cramp	músculo torcido	— a twisted muscle, muscle strain
choque eléctrico	— electrical shock		
deshidratación	— dehydration	parálisis	— paralysis
desmayo	— fainting	picadura de insecto	— insect bite
disparo	— shot	plaga	— plague
emponzoñamiento, envenenamiento	— poisoning	problema abdominal	— abdominal problem
		puñalada	— stabbing or stab wound
epidemia	— epidemic		
espasmo	— spasm	sequía	— drought
golpe	— blow	sofocación	— choking, suffocation
hambre canina	— bad hunger, starvation	shock	— shock
herida	— wound	terremoto	— earthquake
herida de bala	— gunshot wound	tétano	— tetanus
insolación	— sunstroke	tornado	— tornado
intoxicación	— intoxication	traumatismo	— trauma
inundación	— flood	trombosis coronaria	— coronary thrombosis
mal de rabia	— rabies		

2. Spanish names — Nombres hispánicos

		Nombres ingleses — English names	
Abrahán	Leticia	Paul	Phil
Adela	Lucas	Paula	Philip
Bartolomé	Magdalena	Patrick	Randy
Berta	Marcos	Peggy	Rhonda
Camilo	Mateo	Penny	Robin
Diego	Mireya	Perry	Ruth
Filemón	Nancy	Peter	Sara
Haroldo	Omar		
Hildebrando	Orfa		
Iván	Orlando		

3. Useful expressions — Expresiones útiles

traigan ayuda rápidamente	— bring help quickly.
un accidente muy serio	— a very serious accident.
una persona está herida de gravedad	— someone is badly hurt.
está inconsciente por una descarga eléctrica	— He's (She's) unconscious from an electric shock.
el botiquín de primeros auxilios	— first aid kit.
fractura del brazo en la parte de arriba y abajo	— fracture of the upper and lower arm bones.
hay víctimas	— there are victims.
se tragó un alfiler	— He (She) swallowed a pin.
¡Qué susto!	— How frightening!
fue un desastre	— it was a disaster.
tiene una fractura mayor	— He (She) has a bad fracture.

le voy a poner un torniquete	— I am going to put a tourniquet on you.
este es el vendaje	— this is the bandage.
¿Cómo es la herida?	— How serious is the injury?
es un ataque cardíaco	— It's a heart attack.
hay que pedir socorro	— One must ask for help.

4. Idiomatic expressions — Expresiones idiomáticas

Le dieron una puñalada	— He (She) was stabbed.
Por poco se carboniza	— He was almost burned to a crisp.
¡Qué lástima!	— What a pity!
Se ha golpeado	— He (She) has a contusion.
¿Sabes nadar?	— Do you know how to swim?
Tomó alcohol	— He took alcohol.
aspirinas	— aspirin
cianuro	— cyanide
cloro	— bleach
drogas	— drugs
insecticida	— insecticide
lejía	— lye
pastillas para dormir	— sleeping pills
tetracloruro de carbón	— carbon tetrachloride
trementina, aguarrás	— turpentine
tranquilizantes	— tranquilizers
veneno	— poison
Volverse loco	— to go crazy.

5. Some sayings — Algunos dichos

A buen hambre no hay mal pan	— Hunger is the best sauce.
Amor con amor se paga	— One good turn deserves another.
Ayúdate y Dios te ayudará	— God helps those who help themselves.
La caridad empieza por nosotros	— Charity begins at home.
Lo que a uno cura a otro mata	— One man's meat is another man's poison.
No hay que cantar victoria	— Don't whistle before you're out of the woods.
Tal padre, tal hijo	— Like father like son.
Todo lo que brilla no es oro	— All that glitters is not gold.

BILINGUAL PROJECT — PROYECTO BILINGUE

TRANSCRIPTION — TRANSCRIPCION

In the remaining ten lessons of the text the **Preparatory Exercises** have been replaced by **Transcriptions,** all of which obey the same format, although there will be some variation in detail from one lesson to another.

As you can see from the material below, you are given a brief report in English and in Spanish of an incident in someone's life requiring medical treatment. Your first task is to transcribe this brief narration into a truly medical case history by recasting it in medical language and termi-

En las diez lecciones restantes del texto los **ejercicios preparatorios** han sido sustituidos por **transcripciones,** las cuales tienen el mismo formato, aunque habrá algunas variantes de una lección a otra en lo que a los detalles se refiere.

Como lo indica una revisión somera de la materia que se presenta a continuación, a usted, el estudiante, se le proporciona un relato breve tanto en inglés como en español, de un incidente que exige que se preste atención médica a un ser humano. La tarea inicial que tiene usted es la

nology. The net effect should be that of a description written by a professional medical secretary whose intention would be to include it as part of a patient's permanent file or dossier.

Your second task consists in completing the reports as outlined below the narration. These reports would also be drawn up as part of the normal contents of a patient file in a hospital or doctor's office. The format of the final presentation of this project will be explained to you by your Instructor and he will indicate to you the procedure to be followed in doing the transcription and writing the reports.

Again, it is strongly recommended that all students prepare this exercise in both English and Spanish whenever feasible.

de transcribir lo narrado en forma de una verdadera historia clínica, redactándolo de nuevo y usando un lenguaje y terminología médica. El resultado debe lucir como si fuera una descripción hecha por una secretaria médica profesional para ser incluida en la historia médica completa permanente de un paciente.

La segunda tarea consiste en preparar los informes que se indican esquemáticamente después de la narración. Estos informes también se confeccionarán con el objeto de que entren a formar parte de la historia médica permanente de un paciente en el archivo de algún hospital o médico particular. El formato de la presentación final de este proyecto se lo explicará a usted el profesor de la materia, quién le puntualizará también el procedimiento a seguir al redactar la transcripción y los informes. De nuevo, se recomienda con gran énfasis que todos los estudiantes preparen este ejercicio en ambos idiomas, siempre que sea factible hacerlo así.

NAME — NOMBRE _____

ADDRESS — DIRECCION _____

SITUATION — SITUACION _____

This 17 year-old girl was seriously injured in an automobile accident and rushed to the medical center. She was given initial life saving treatment in the shock-trauma unit. Various X-ray studies were done to evaluate the extent of her injuries and she was brought to surgery. Her convalescence was lengthy, but her recovery was good, and she was discharged several weeks after admission.

Esta joven de 17 años fue herida gravemente en un accidente automovilístico y fue llevada de emergencia al centro médico. Le dieron un tratamiento inicial para evitar el shock y salvarle la vida. Le hicieron varios exámenes radiográficos para evaluar las heridas y la llevaron a cirugía. Su convalescencia fue morosa pero su recuperación fue buena y la dieron de alta varias semanas después de ser admitida.

SEQUENCE OF REPORTS   —   ORDEN DE LOS INFORMES

A—1

History and Physical Exam
Historia y examen físico

Completed _____

Terminado _____

A—2

X-ray Report
Informe radiológico

Completed _____

Terminado _____

A—3

Surgical Record
Informe quirúrgico

Completed _____

Terminado _____

A—4

Clinical Resume
Resumen clínico

Completed _____

Terminado _____

EXERCISES — EJERCICIOS

(Students learning Spanish — Estudiantes de español)

A. Translate into Spanish

1. He just finished his composition. ....

2. I fell and broke my arm. ....

3. Manuel has twenty books. ....

4. He has a brother who is a doctor. ....

5. The nurse is at the emergency room. ....

B. Translate the English words in each sentence.

1. (These) pacientes están más enfermos que (those). ....

2. ¿Quién te contó (that) historia? ....

3. (Those) medicinas son más fuertes que (these). ....

4. (This) tratamiento es muy efectivo. ....

5. Me gusta mucho (that — farther away) país. ....

C. Make a list (in Spanish) of the items that should be included in a first aid kit.

....

....

D. Explain (in Spanish) an accident that you have witnessed.

....

....

....

E. Write six sentences (in Spanish) using the forms of "acabar de" in each sentence.

1. ....   4. ....

2. ....   5. ....

3. ....   6. ....

F. Answer in Spanish.

1. ¿Cuántos accidentes ha presenciado usted? ....

2. ¿Qué hace usted cuando nada en un lago? ....

3. ¿Por qué son importantes los botes salvavidas? ....

4. ¿Qué se debe hacer cuando se recibe una mordedura de serpiente? ......

....

5. ¿A quién llamaría usted en caso de un envenenamiento? ....

EJERCICIOS — EXERCISES

(Estudiantes de inglés — Students learning English)

A. Cambie las siguientes oraciones al plural.

1. This is my doctor. ....
2. This notebook is mine; that one is yours. ....
3. That pen over there is yours. ....
4. That is a very small hospital. ....
5. This exercise is difficult. ....

B. Tradúzcase al inglés.

1. Me caí y me quebré el brazo. ....
2. Peter tiene esos papeles. ....
3. El tiene un hermano que es doctor. ....
4. El camión chocó con una camioneta. ....
5. Hubo muchos heridos y varios muertos. ....

C. Escriba cuatro oraciones usando to have just y algunos de los modismos que ya conoce.

1. ....   3. ....
2. ....   4. ....

D. Haga una lista de cosas que debe una persona tener en un botiquín de primeros auxilios.

....
....

E. Explique algún accidente que Ud. haya presenciado; haga mención de la intervención de la policía.

....
....
....

F. Conteste las siguientes preguntas en inglés con oraciones completas.

1. When did you see an accident? ....
2. What would you do if a person were drowning in a swimming pool? ....
3. What is the number of the Fire Department? ....
4. Where is the Rescue Squad? ....
5. Where is the Police Station? ....

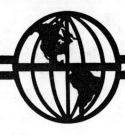

LABORATORY EXAMINATIONS
EXAMENES DE LABORATORIO

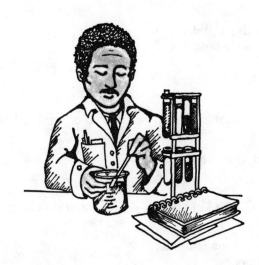

VOCABULARY — VOCABULARIO

A. Medical — Médico

albumina	— albumin	laboratorio	— laboratory
análisis	— analysis	metabolismo	— metabolism
coagulación	— coagulation	microscopio	— microscope
coágulo	— coagulated blood	orina	— urine
costra	— scab	técnico	— technician (lab technician)
esputo	— sputum, saliva, spit		
excremento, materia fecal	— excrement, stool	tubo	— tube
		unto	— smear
instrumento	— instrument	urinálisis, análisis de orina	— urinalysis
jeringa, jeringuilla	— syringe, hypodermic needle		

B. General

además	— besides	investigación sobre la leucemia	— leukemia research
cianuro	— cyanide		
clase	— kind	medir	— to measure
chancro	— chancre	negativos	— negatives
dieta sin sal	— salt free diet	pellizcar	— to pinch
doloroso	— painful	pinchar	— to pierce, puncture
enfermedades venéreas	— venereal diseases	positivo	— positive
examen	— test, examination	prueba	— test
frecuentemente	— frequently	rutina, rutinario (a)	— routine
gonorrea	— gonorrhea	sífilis	— syphilis
inflamarse	— to become inflamed	síntoma	— symptom
ingle	— groin	tantos (as)	— as many, so many

CONVERSATION — CONVERSACION

A. Gabriel Jacobo visits Dr. Collins; his son Isaías does the translating.

Gabriel Jacobo visita al Dr. Collins; su hijo Isaías le hace la traducción.

Gabriel	— Buenos días, doctor.	
Dr. Collins	— Buenos días, Mr. Jacobo... How long has it been since your last visit?	*Good morning, Mr. Jacobo... ¿cuánto hace que no me visita?*
Isaías	— El doctor quiere saber cuánto tiempo hace que no lo visitas.	
Gabriel	— Un par de años.	*A couple of years.*
Isaías	— Two years.	
Dr. Collins	— Today I'll send him to the laboratory.	*Hoy lo enviaré al laboratorio.*
Isaías	— Hoy te enviará al laboratorio.	
Gabriel	— ¿Para qué?	*What for?*
Dr. Collins	— The technician will take samples for some tests.	*El laboratorista le tomará muestras para algunos exámenes.*
Isaías	— El laboratorista te tomará muestras para algunos exámenes.	
Gabriel	— ¿Qué clase de muestras?	*What kind of samples?*
Isaías	— What kind of samples?	
Dr. Collins	— Samples of urine, blood, saliva and stool.	*Muestras de orina, sangre, saliva y excremento.*
Isaías	— Muestras de orina, sangre, saliva y excremento.	
Gabriel	— ¿Por qué tantas?	*Why so many?*
Isaías	— Why so many?	
Dr. Collins	— Tell him not to worry. They are routine examinations.	*Dígale que no se preocupe. Son exámenes de rutina.*
Isaías	— Son exámenes de rutina.	
Dr. Collins	— Here is the written order.	*Aquí está la orden por escrito.*
Isaías	— Aquí está la orden por escrito.	
Gabriel	— Dale las gracias, y vamos al laboratorio.	*Tell him thank you, and let's go to the lab.*
Isaías	— Thank you, Dr. Collins.	
Dr. Collins	— Tell him I'll let him know about the results.	*Dígale que ya le avisaré acerca de los resultados.*
Gabriel	— Gracias.	
Isaías	— Good by.	
Dr. Collins	— By.	

GRAMMATICAL HINTS — APUNTES GRAMATICALES

A. Hacer is used in different idiomatic ways.

1. To express **please:**

Haga el favor de cerrar la boca — Please close your mouth.
Haga el favor de abrir la puerta — Please open the door.

2. With a period of time it means **ago:**

Me visitó hace cinco años   — He visited me five years ago.
Hace cuatro semanas que empecé a   — I began to study Spanish four weeks ago.
    estudiar español.

3. To express an act that began in the past and is still going on in the present:

Hace cinco años que no me visita   — He hasn't visited me for five years.
Hace cuatro semanas que estudio   — I have been studying Spanish for four
    español.   weeks.

4. When dealing with the **weather:**

Hace frío — It is cold;   Hace calor — It is hot;   Hace fresco — It is cool.

B. Supposed to

1. La frase **supposed to,** que ocurre frecuentemente en inglés, se usa para mostrar una obligación que tiene que cumplir el sujeto, y a veces para expresar expectación.
    e.g. John is supposed to work today   — Juan debe trabajar hoy.
        Everybody is supposed to come   — Todos deben (se supone que van a) venir.

2. Esta frase verbal, **supposed to,** se usa solamente con el presente y el pretérito.

C. Used to

1. Esta frase verbal corresponde al imperfecto de indicativo en español, porque se refiere a una acción del pasado pero que continúa por un tiempo indefinido.
Would tiene la misma función que **used to** en esta construcción.
    e.g. The patient used to smoke — El paciente solía fumar (es decir, fumó por un tiempo en el pasado pero dejó de fumar).
        I used to work at the hospital; but now I work at the university —
        Trabajaba en el hospital; pero ahora trabajo en la universidad.

2. No hay que confundir **used to** con **to be used to,** que significa estar acostumbrado a algo. El **to** en esta frase es una preposición y por lo tanto está seguido por un sustantivo o un gerundio.
    e.g. I am used to wearing glasses — Estoy acostumbrado a usar anteojos.

D. The preterit form of a verb is used to indicate the **definite** happening of something in the past. It implies that there was a beginning and an end. The time limit is expressed by the context.

The imperfect of a verb is used to indicate repeated or habitual actions in the past. The English equivalent is generally expressed by **used to** to show a progressive construction. The action of the imperfect form is seen as continuing over a period of time and its probable beginning or end is ignored.

E. Imperfect indicative

1. The conjugation of all verbs in the imperfect indicative goes like this:

Habl**aba** — I was talking, talked   com**ía**   — I was eating, ate
habl**abas**   com**ías**
habl**aba**   com**ía**
habl**ábamos**   com**íamos**
habl**aban**   com**ían**

2. There are only three irregular verbs in the imperfect indicative:

ser: era, eras, era, éramos, eran.
ir :   iba, ibas, iba, íbamos, iban.
ver: veía, veías, veía, veíamos, veían.

3. Uses of the imperfect:

a) Duration in past time, the end of which is not implied.
Cuando **vivía** en Madrid **iba** todos los días a la universidad.

b) Description in the past.
Era un hogar feliz...

c) Continuing action (or state), which may be interrupted (by a verb in the preterit).
Cuando el paciente **salía llegó** el doctor.

d) Time of day
Eran las cinco cuando el técnico vino a trabajar.

e) Indirect discourse in the past, which has replaced a present indirect discourse or direct discourse.
Ella dijo que todos los exámenes **eran** negativos. (Dice que todos **son** negativos).

CONVERSATION — CONVERSACION

B. Débora who works in the lab, meets Patricia, who is a nurse for Dr. Gates; Amelia does the translating.

Débora, que trabaja en el laboratorio, se encuentra con Patricia, una enfermera del Dr. Gates; Amelia les hace la traducción.

Débora — ¿Dónde estabas ayer, Patricia?

Where were you yesterday, Patricia?

Amelia — Débora is wondering where you were yesterday.

Débora se pregunta dónde estabas ayer.

Patricia — Yesterday was my day off, and I went shopping.

Ayer fue mi día libre y me fui de compras.

Amelia — Tenía el día libre y se fue de compras.

Patricia — What did you do yesterday?

¿Qué hiciste ayer?

Amelia — ¿Qué hiciste ayer?

Débora — Ayer me tocó hacer varios exámenes.

Yesterday I had to do several examinations.

Amelia — She had to do several examinations.

Patricia — What type?

¿Qué clase?

Amelia — ¿Qué clase?

Débora — Le aplicamos el examen del conejo a una señora.

We gave the rabbit test to a lady.

Amelia — She gave the rabbit test to a lady.

Patricia — To see if she was pregnant?

¿Para ver si estaba embarazada?

Amelia — ¿Para ver si estaba embarazada?

Débora — Sí. Después tuvimos que hacer un recuento globular, medir la albúmina y medir el metabolismo de otros pacientes.

Yes, and afterwards, we had to do a blood count, measure the albumin, and measure the metabolism of other patients.

Amelia — Yes. Afterwards, they had to do a blood count, measure the albumin, and measure the metabolism of other patients.

Patricia — How is your work today?

¿Cómo estás de trabajo hoy?

Amelia — ¿Cómo estás de trabajo hoy?

Débora — Más o menos lo mismo.

About the same.

Patricia — Such is life.

Así es la vida.

Amelia — Así es la vida.

Débora — Sí, así es la vida.

GRAMMATICAL HINTS — APUNTES GRAMATICALES

F. Otros adjetivos

Much se usa con sustantivos en singular, particularmente cuando se refiere a una cantidad indefinida, la cual se puede medir, pero no contar (mass nouns).
e.g. much sugar — mucha azúcar;   much work — mucho trabajo.

Much se emplea generalmente en oraciones negativas: I don't have much money.
En oraciones positivas se usa a **lot of** or **a great deal of:** He has a lot of money.

Many se usa con sustantivos en plural (count nouns).
e.g. The hospital has many beds — El hospital tiene muchas camas (se puede contar el número de camas que hay).

Less se usa con sustantivos singulares (mass nouns: no se pueden contar).
e.g. less blood — menos sangre; less time — menos tiempo.

Few se usa con sustantivos en plural así como **many,** pero en sentido contrario.
(count nouns: se puede contar el número de items).
e.g. I have few books — Tengo pocos libros.

CONVERSATION — CONVERSACION

C. The doctor, the patient and the interpreter.

El doctor, el paciente y un intérprete.

Doctor — ¿Tomó la medicina que le receté?

Did you take the medicine I prescribed?

Interpreter — Did you take the medicine he prescribed?

Patient	— I am still taking it.		*Todavía la estoy tomando.*
Interpreter	— Todavía la está tomando.		
Doctor	— ¿Cómo está su apetito?		*How is your appetite?*
Interpreter	— How is your appetite?		
Patient	— Better, doctor. Now I am hungry more often, and I feel more like eating the meals.		*Mejor, doctor. Ahora tengo más hambre y como las comidas con más apetito.*
Interpreter	— Se siente mejor. Ahora tiene más hambre y come las comidas con más apetito.		
Doctor	— Como se siente mejor le voy a cambiar la receta, y dígale que quiero verlo el próximo miércoles para ver cómo sigue.		*Since he's feeling better, I am going to change his prescription, and tell him I would like to see him next Wednesday to see how he feels.*
Interpreter	— Since you're feeling better, he is going to change the prescription, but he wants to see you next Wednesday.		
Patient	— Good!		*¡Bueno!*
Interpreter	— Good!		
Doctor	— ¡Bueno!		

Cells — Células

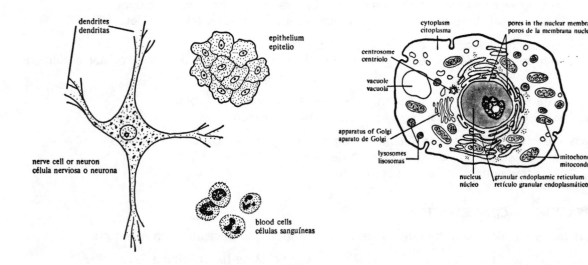

dendrites
dendritas

epithelium
epitelio

nerve cell or neuron
célula nerviosa o neurona

blood cells
células sanguíneas

cytoplasm
citoplasma

pores in the nuclear membrane
poros de la membrana nuclear

centrosome
centriolo

vacuole
vacuola

apparatus of Golgi
aparato de Golgi

lysosomes
lisosomas

nucleus
núcleo

mitochondria
mitocondrias

granular endoplasmic reticulum
retículo granular endoplasmático

THE MUSCLES — LOS MUSCULOS

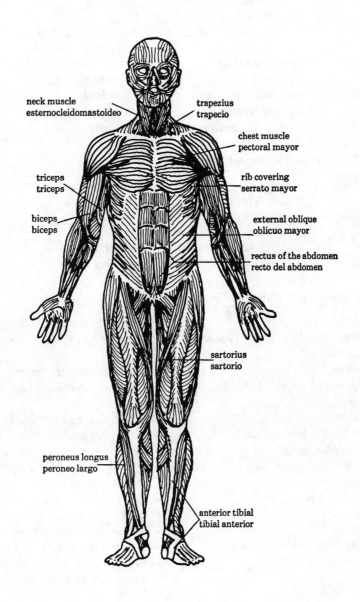

neck muscle
esternocleidomastoideo

trapezius
trapecio

chest muscle
pectoral mayor

triceps
triceps

rib covering
serrato mayor

biceps
bíceps

external oblique
oblicuo mayor

rectus of the abdomen
recto del abdomen

sartorius
sartorio

peroneus longus
peroneo largo

anterior tibial
tibial anterior

ADDITIONAL INFORMATION — INFORMACION ADICIONAL

1. Specialists — Especialistas

anestesista	— anesthetist, anesthesiologist	ginecólogo	— gynecologist
		homeópata	— homeopathist
bacteriólogo	— bacteriologist	internista	— internist
cardiólogo	— cardiologist	masajista	— masseur, masseuse
cirujano dentista	— dental surgeon	médico cirujano	— surgeon
dentista	— dentist	médico partero, tocólogo	— obstetrician
dermatólogo	— dermatologist		
gastroenterólogo	— gastroenterologist	neurólogo	— neurologist

oculista, oftalmólogo — ophtalmologist, oculist, eye doctor
optometrista, optómetro — optician, optometrist, oculist
ortodontista — orthodontist
ortopedista — orthopedist
otólogo — aurist
otorrinolaringólogo — otolaryngologist (ear, nose, and throat specialist)

patólogo — pathologist
pediatra — pediatrician, pediatrist
podiatra, pedicuro, cirujano callista — podiatrist, foot doctor
psyquiatra o siquiatra — psychiatrist
quiropráctico — chiropractor
radiólogo — radiologist
taxidermista — taxidermist
urólogo — urologist

2. Bacteriological terms — Términos bactereológicos

bacilo — bacillus
bacteria — bacterium
coco, micrococo — coccus, micrococcus
diplococo — diplococcus
espirilo — spirillum
espiroqueto (a) — spirochete

estafilococo — staphylococcus
estreptococo — streptococcus
miocardio — miocardium, heart muscle
sarcitis — sarcitis, miositis
vibrión — vibrio

3. Useful expressions — Expresiones útiles

¿Cuánto pesa Ud.? — How much do you weigh?
¿Tiene problemas con el corazón? (¿una deficiencia cardíaca?) — Do you have heart trouble?
¿Sufre de diabetes? — Do you have diabetes?
¿Sufre de alta presión? (¿tiene la tensión sanguínea alta?) — Do you have high blood pressure?
¿Qué fue lo último que comió Ud.? — What did you eat last?
Necesita seguir las órdenes médicas — You have to follow the doctor's directions.
¿Tiene Ud. la orden escrita? — Do you have the written order?
Vamos a hacerle un examen para ver si tiene azúcar en la sangre — We are going to give you a test for sugar in the blood.
Hacer un conteo, un recuento — To take a count.
Tomar un unto — To take a smear.
Medir la albúmina — To measure the albumin.
Necesita un reconocimiento médico — You need a physical examination.
Favor de cerrar el puño — Please make a fist (close your fist).
Favor de abrir la mano — Please open your hand, fist.

4. Idiomatic expressions — Expresiones idiomáticas

Allí mismo — right there
El cielo no está claro, despejado — The sky is not clear.
¿Qué tiempo hace hoy? — How's the weather today?
Hace buen tiempo — It's nice, nice weather.
Hace calor — It's hot.
Hace fresco — It's cool.
Hace frío — It's cold.
Hace sol — It's sunny.
Hace viento — It's windy.
Tener que — to have to.

BILINGUAL PROJECT — PROYECTO BILINGUE

TRANSCRIPTION — TRANSCRIPCION

Complete the following reports along with the completed transcription. (See pp. 107-108).

Prepare la siguiente transcripción y termine los informes adjuntos. (Vea pág. 107-108).

NAME — NOMBRE: _____

ADDRESS — DIRECCION: _____

SITUATION — SITUACION:

This 40 year-old male was found unconscious in the men's room at his place of work and taken to the hospital in an ambulance. He was examined and a diagnosis of diabetic coma was made. He was seen in consultation by a specialist. X-ray tests were taken. He responded to treatment and was discharged.

Este señor de 40 años de edad fue encontrado en estado inconsciente en el baño (sanitario) de hombres donde trabaja y fue llevado al hospital en ambulancia. Fue examinado y se le diagnosticó una coma diabética. Fue visto por un especialista consultante. Se le tomaron radiografías. Respondió al tratamiento y fue dado de alta.

SEQUENCE OF REPORTS — ORDEN DE LOS INFORMES

A—1

History and Physical Exam
Historia y examen físico

Completed _____

Terminado _____

A—2

Consultant's Report
Informe del consultante

Completed _____

Terminado _____

A—3

X-ray Report
Informe radiológico

Completed _____

Terminado _____

A—4

Clinical Resumé
Resumen clínico

Completed _____

Terminado _____

EXERCISES — EJERCICIOS

(Students learning Spanish — Estudiantes de español)

A. Translate into Spanish.

1. Today it is cold. ....

2. The lab technician is very nice. ....

3. Please open your mouth. ....

4. I came to school two weeks ago. ....

5. I have to take some medical examinations. ....

B. Fill in the blank in each of the following sentences by selecting the appropriate form in parentheses.

1. _____ cinco años que visité España. (hago, hace, haga)

2. Trabajan en _____ hospital. (este, esta, estos)

3. Hoy _____ mucho calor. (haz, haga, hace)

4. Ayer Juanito _____ de la bicicleta. (calló, cayó, se cayó)

5. El paciente _____ al laboratorio. (voy, vas, va)

C. Answer in Spanish.

1. ¿Por qué es importante la medicina? ....

2. ¿Qué se hace en el laboratorio? ....

3. ¿Para qué sirve el cloro en el agua potable? ....

4. ¿Quién es el laboratorista de su hospital? ....

5. ¿Cuándo fue la última vez que recibió usted un examen completo de laboratorio?
   ....

D. Fill in each blank with the proper form of each verb in the imperfect.

1. La enferma (estar) _____ en el hospital.

2. Anteriormente la enfermera (trabajar) _____ en una clínica.

3. El dijo que el doctor siempre (llegar) _____ a tiempo.

4. Los exámenes (resultar) _____ siempre negativos.

5. ¿Qué (tener) _____ el paciente?

E. Fill in the blanks with the proper form of the verb by choosing either the preterit or imperfect form.

1. Anoche el enfermero (trabajar) _____ en el laboratorio.

2. Luis (pagar) _____ todas sus deudas y (salir) _____ del país.

3. (ser) _____ las cuatro cuando (llegar) _____ el paciente.

4. El trabajador social (venir) _____ todas las tardes a su casa.

5. El radiólogo (hacer) _____ las radiografías.

F. Write a short composition describing the work of a lab technician.

....

....

....

....

EJERCICIOS — EXERCISES

(Estudiantes de inglés — Students learning English)

A. Llene los espacios vacíos con el adjetivo correspondiente.

1. The university has _____ (muchos) students this year.
2. The clinic has _____ (pocas) patients this year.
3. The technician has _____ (menos) work this year.
4. We need _____ (mucha) sugar.
5. He has (pocos) _____ patients.

B. Traduzca al inglés.

1. Yo iba al trabajo todos los días. ....
2. Debemos hacer nuestra tarea. ....
3. El paciente está acostumbrado a tomar una siesta. ....
4. ¿Tiene Ud. mucha paciencia? ....
5. Hay pocos pacientes en este hospital. ....

C. Escriba una composición corta en que describa el trabajo y las responsabilidades de un técnico de laboratorio.

....
....
....
....
....

D. Conteste en inglés.

1. What do you do to improve your appetite? ....
2. Why is medicine so important? ....
3. What is the most important medicine for cancer? ....
4. What is the name of the lab technician? ....
5. What can you do to get rid of a headache? ....

E. Escriba cuatro oraciones usando expresiones idiomáticas.

1. ....   3. ....
2. ....   4. ....

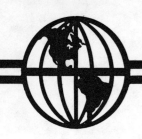

COMMUNICABLE DISEASES
ENFERMEDADES CONTAGIOSAS

VOCABULARY — VOCABULARIO

A. Medical — Médico

evitar contagio	— to void infection	resfriado	— cold
influenza, catarro	— heavy cold, influenza, flu	sarampión alemán	— German measles
		tétano	— tetanus
inmunización	— immunization	tónico	— tonic
laxante, purgante	— laxative, purgative	tuberculosis	— tuberculosis, TB
paludismo, malaria	— malaria	vacunar	— to vaccinate
poliomielitis, parálisis infantil	— poliomyelitis, infatile paralysis, "polio"	viruela	— smallpox

B. General

aeropuerto	— airport	itinerario	— itinerary, routing, schedule of travel
agua	— water		
azafata, aeromoza	— stewardess, airline hostess	listo	— ready
		pasaporte	— passport
compañero	— companion	peligroso	— dangerous, hazardous
desinfectar	— to disinfect		
epidemia	— epidemic	pescador	— fisherman
expuesto	— exposed	regañar	— to scold
fotografía, foto	— photograph, photo, picture	suficiente	— enough, sufficient
		viaje	— trip
fumar	— to smoke	vuelo	— flight

CONVERSATION — CONVERSACION

A. Dionisio and his wife, Lisa, visit Dr. Castle.   Dionisio y su esposa Lisa visitan al Dr. Castle

Doctor	— Good morning, may I help you?	*Buenos días, ¿en qué podemos servirles?*
Lisa	— My husband needs help.	*Mi esposo necesita ayuda.*
Doctor	— What's his problem?	*¿Cuál es su problema?*
Lisa	— One of his friends from work has tuberculosis.	*Uno de sus compañeros de trabajo tiene tuberculosis.*
Doctor	— Where does he work?	*¿Dónde trabaja él?*
Lisa	— He is a fisherman.	*Es pescador.*
Doctor	— Ask him how he knows his friend has TB?	*Pregúntele que cómo sabe que su amigo tiene tuberculosis?*

Lisa	— ¿Cómo sabes que tu amigo tiene tuberculosis?	
Dionisio	— Porque tose mucho.	*Because he coughs a lot.*
Lisa	— Because he coughs a lot.	
Doctor	— Does he smoke a lot?	*¿Fuma mucho?*
Lisa	— ¿Fuma mucho?	
Dionisio	— El no fuma.	*He doesn't smoke.*
Doctor	— Tell him not to worry. Let's wait and see what the X-ray photo says.	*Dígale que no se preocupe. Vamos a esperar a ver que dice la radiografía.*
Lisa	— No te preocupes. Vamos a esperar los resultados de la radiografía.	
Doctor	— In the meantime we'll give him a vaccination. The vaccination will help prevent infection. Tell him to try to avoid any direct contact with his friend.	*Mientras tanto le vamos a poner una vacuna. La vacuna le ayudará a prevenir el contagio. Dígale que procure evitar cualquier contacto con su amigo.*
Lisa	— Te van a poner una vacuna. Pero el doctor quiere que evites cualquier contacto con tu amigo.	
Dionisio	— Bueno.	
Lisa	— He agrees.	*El está de acuerdo.*
Doctor	— All right.	

GRAMMATICAL HINTS — APUNTES GRAMATICALES

A. Object pronouns in Spanish

1. The table of object pronouns is as follows:

Direct	Indirect	Prepositional
me	me	mí
te	te	ti
la, lo (le)	le	él, ella, Ud.
nos	nos	nosotros, (as)
los, las	les	ellos, ellas, Uds.

2. Object pronouns regularly precede the verb.
Leo **el libro** — **lo** leo.
Miran **los programas** — **los** miran.

B. Formas objetivas del pronombre en inglés

1. Las formas objetivas del prenombre son más fáciles en inglés que en español. Estas formas sirven como complementos directos, indirectos y circunstanciales. Estos pronombres son:

me	us
you	you
him, her, it	them

2. Estos pronombres van después del verbo.

    e.g. We saw **her** at the clinic — **La** vimos en la clínica.

       He gave **us** the medicine — **Nos** dio la medicina.

       He gave **it** to **me** — **Me lo** (**la**) dio.

       Mary studies English with **him** — Mary estudia inglés con **él**.

CONVERSATION — CONVERSACION (Cont.)

B. Elena Bermudez takes her son to the doctor, her neighbor Lori goes with her to interpret for her.

Elena Bermúdez lleva a su hijo donde el doctor; su vecina Lori va con ella para ayudarle como intérprete.

Elena — Buenos días, doctor.

Good morning, doctor.

Doctor — Good morning, what can I do for you?

Buenos días, ¿en qué puedo servirle?

Lori — ¿En qué puede servirte?

What can he do for you?

Elena — Dile que en nuestro vecindario hay una epidemia de viruela, y no quiero que mi hijo se enferme.

Tell him that in our neighborhood there is a smallpox epidemic and I don't want my son to get sick.

Lori — There is a smallpox epidemic in our neighborhood and she doesn't want her son to get sick.

Doctor — Is her son here?

¿Está su hijo aquí?

Lori — Yes, he is in the waiting room.

Sí, está en la sala de espera.

Doctor — Bring him in, I am going to give him a vaccination.

Tráigalo, le voy a poner una vacuna.

Lori — Voy a traer a Jaime. El doctor le va a poner una vacuna.

I am going to bring Jaime in. The doctor is going to give him a vaccination.

Elena — Pregúntele si puede darle otras vacunas al mismo tiempo.

Ask him if he can give him other vaccinations at the same time.

Lori — Can you give him other vaccinations?

Doctor — Such as?

¿Como cuáles?

Elena — Contra el polio, el tétano y el sarampión.

Against polio, tetanus, and the measles.

Lori — Against polio, tetanus and the measles.

Doctor — One vaccine is sufficient for today.

Una vacuna es suficiente por ahora.

Lori — Una vacuna es suficiente por ahora.

Elena — Muy bien.

All right.

Lori — All right.

Doctor — Good.

GRAMMATICAL HINTS — APUNTES GRAMATICALES (Cont.)

C. More object pronouns

1. The indirect object precedes the direct object. If both pronominal objects are in the third person, the indirect object **le** (**les**) becomes **se** (not to be confused with the reflexive **se**).
   Escribo **un poema** para **ella. Se lo** escribo.
   Me traen las medicinas. **Me las** traen.

2. Object pronouns follow and are attached to infinitives, present participles and affirmative imperatives.
   Vamos a lavarle **la herida.** Vamos a lavar**la.**
   ¡Tome el jarabe! Tóme**lo.**
   Ellos están buscando **la medicina.** Están buscándo**la.**
   La enfermera está poniendo **una inyección al paciente.** Está poniéndo**sela.**

3. A written accent is placed over the syllable originally stressed in affirmative commands and present participles.
   Cóma**sela.**   No **se la** coma.   Están ofreciéndo**noslo.**

4. When an infinitive or present participle is used immediately after another verb, the object pronouns may precede or follow.

   Estamos buscándo**la**   or   **la** estamos buscando.
   Van a escribir**los**   or   **los** van a escribir.

D. The prepositional object pronouns are used:

1. As the object of a preposition
   El doctor vacunó a **él,** a **mí,** a **ti,** a **nosotros.**
   (With **con** there is an exception in the first and second person singular which are written: con**migo,** con**tigo**).

2. After verbs of motion.
   Los pacientes volverán a **mí.**

E. There was, there were.

1. Como ya se había explicado en lecciones anteriores, **hay** se traduce **there is** para la forma singular y **there are** para el plural.
   e.g. There is a hospital over there — hay un hospital por allí.
   There are many patients — hay muchos pacientes.

2. La forma pasada **había, hubo,** se traduce: **there was** para el singular y **there were** para el plural.
   e.g. There was a book here — había un libro aquí.
   There were many books — había muchos libros.

F. Más verbos auxiliares

1. Como ya se había explicado en lecciones anteriores, **to have to** significa **tener que.**

2. **Should** y **ought** seguidos por un infinitivo expresan en forma suave un deber o una obligación.
   e.g. You should see a doctor   — debe ver a un doctor.
   You ought to see a doctor   — (nótese que **ought** está seguido siempre por **to**)

3. **Must** es otro verbo defectivo que se usa con el infinitivo para expresar:

   a) gran necesidad o mandato
   e.g. We must finish this work today — debemos terminar este trabajo hoy.
   You must call the doctor at once — debe llamar al doctor en seguida.

b) gran posibilidad (con el verbo **to be**)
   e.g. This must be the nurse — debe (debe de) ser la enfermera.
       He must be sick — debe (debe de) estar enfermo.

CONVERSATION — CONVERSACION (Cont.)

C. El Dr. Ramiro Castellanos está planeando tomar unas vacaciones con su familia y le pide a su secretaria que haga los arreglos necesarios.

Dr. Ramiro Castellanos is planning to take a vacation with his family and asks his secretarty to make the necessary arrangements.

Castellanos — Señorita, ¿está todo listo?

Miss, is everything ready?

Secretaria — Todavía no.

Not yet.

Castellanos — ¿Qué tenemos que hacer?

What do we have to do?

Secretaria — Tiene que tomarse una foto con su familia para conseguir luego el pasaporte.

You must have a picture taken with your family to get the passaport.

Castellanos — ¿Cuánto tiempo se demora el pasaporte?

How long does it take to get the passport?

Secretaria — Unos diez días.

About ten days.

Castellanos — Y después ¿qué tenemos que hacer?

Then what do we have to do?

Secretaria — Tienen que vacunarse todos.

Then everyone needs to get vaccinated.

Castellanos — ¿Y después?

Then what?

Secretaria — Después es el viaje.

Then you'll go on your trip.

Castellanos — ¿Cuál es entonces el itinerario?

What is the schedule?

Secretaria — Permítame confirmar con la agencia de viajes.

Let me check with the Travel Agency.

Castellanos — Bueno.

Secretaria — This is Dr. Ramiro Castellanos' secretary, do you have his schedule ready?

Habla la secretaria del Dr. Ramiro Castellanos ¿tienen ya listo su itinerario?

Agencia — Dr. Castellanos and his family will leave next month on Wednesday the 14th at 1:30 p.m., TWA flight No. 846 to New York, and from New York they will fly to Paris. The rest of the trip will be by train.

Secretaria — Ud. y su familia saldrán por TWA, vuelo No. 846 el próximo mes, el miércoles 14 a la 1:30 p.m. a Nueva York, de Nueva York volarán a París. El resto del viaje será por tren.

Castellanos — ¡Magnífico!

Great!

ADDITIONAL INFORMATION — INFORMACIÓN ADICIONAL

1. Other contagious diseases — Otras enfermedades contagiosas

cólera	— cholera	hepatitis	— hepatitis
difteria	— diphtheria	paperas	— mumps
disentería	— dysentery	pleuresía	— pleurisy
escarlatina	— scarlet fever	pulmonía	— pneumonia
fiebre amarilla	— yellow fever	tifus, tifo	— typhus
fiebre tifoidea	— typhoid fever	tos ferina o convulsiva	— whooping cough

2. El canal alimenticio — alimentary canal

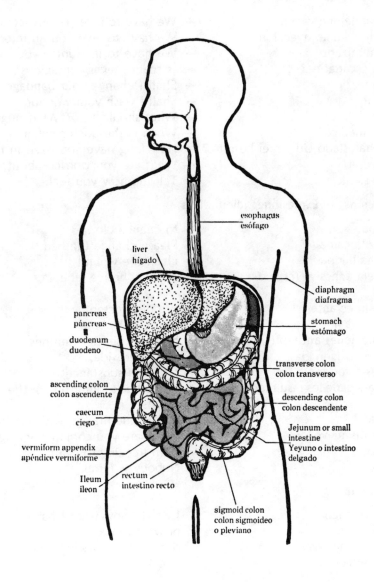

esophagus
esófago

liver
hígado

diaphragm
diafragma

pancreas
páncreas

stomach
estómago

duodenum
duodeno

transverse colon
colon transverso

ascending colon
colon ascendente

descending colon
colon descendente

caecum
ciego

Jejunum or small
intestine
Yeyuno o intestino
delgado

vermiform appendix
apéndice vermiforme

Ileum
ileon

rectum
intestino recto

sigmoid colon
colon sigmoideo
o pleviano

3. Spanish Last Names

		Nombres ingleses	
Alarcón	del Valle	Steve	Tina
Altamirano	Echeverría	Tammy	Todd
Bermúdez	Londoño	Ted	Tom
Caraveo	Narváez	Terri	Valerie
Castellanos	Nieto	Terry	Vicky
Cervantes	Núñez	Theresa	Walter
Corona	Pacheco	Thomas	Wendy
de Angel	Quiroga	Tim	Yvonne
de la Torre	Vásquez		

4. Useful expressions — Expresiones útiles

Tenemos que ponerle una vacuna — We have to give you a vaccination.
Tenemos que ponerle una inyección — We have to give you an injection.
Tenemos que inmunizarlo — We have to immunize you.
¿Es contagiosa la escarlatina? — Is scarlet fever contagious?
¿Le cambio la venda? — Shall I change your bandage?
¿Le lavo la herida? — Shall I wash your wound?
¿Qué debo hacer? — What should I do? What ought I to do?
¿Cuándo viene el médico? — When is the doctor coming?
¿Cuánto tiempo ha estado Ud. en el hospital? — How long have you been in the hospital?
¿De qué se preocupa? — What are you worried about?
Dígame cómo se siente — Tell me how you feel.

5. Idiomatic expressions — Expresiones idiomáticas

Cambiarse de ropa — to change clothes
Favor de cambiar la cama — Please change the bed.
    limpiar la herida — clean the wound
    poner tela adhesiva (espara- — apply adhesive tape
    drapo)
    usar desinfectante — use disinfectant
    esterilizar la llaga — sterilize the sore
    traer soluciones antisépticas — bring antiseptic solutions
    traer agua oxigenada — bring peroxide
    tomar esta sustancia — take this substance
Venga mañana para darle los resultados — Come back tomorrow for the results.

¿Qué le pasa a Ud.? — What's the matter (with you)?
¿Cuándo regresas de nuevo? — When are you coming back again?
Me muero de frío — I am freezing to death.
Nadie es inmune — Nobody is inmune.

6. Proverb — Proverbio

Yo no sé lo que yo tengo
ni sé lo que me hace falta,
que siempre espero una cosa
que no sé cómo se llama.

I don't know what I have
or what I lack
or the name of what it is
I seek.

7. The ear — El oído

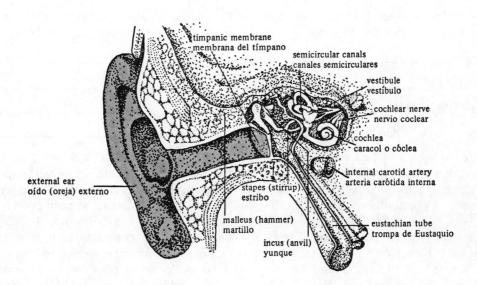

timpanic membrane
membrana del tímpano

semicircular canals
canales semicirculares

vestibule
vestíbulo

cochlear nerve
nervio coclear

cochlea
caracol o cóclea

internal carotid artery
arteria carótida interna

external ear
oído (oreja) externo

stapes (stirrup)
estribo

malleus (hammer)
martillo

incus (anvil)
yunque

eustachian tube
trompa de Eustaquio

8. Useful expressions while traveling — Expresiones útiles mientras se viaja

viaje de negocios	— business trip
hacer reservación en el hotel	— to make a hotel reservation
el gerente	— the manager
hacer bajar el equipaje	— to have one's luggage taken (brought) down
¿Hay una carta para mí?	— Do I have any mail?
Despiérteme temprano	— Call (wake) me early.
Toque el timbre una vez	— Ring the bell once.
Prepáreme el baño	— Have (get) my bath ready.
agua fría, caliente	— cold, hot water
deseo un guía que hable inglés	— I want a guide who speaks English.
¿Ha preguntado alguien por mí?	— Has anyone asked for me?
No vale la pena	— It's not worthwhile. It isn't worth the trouble.

BILINGUAL PROJECT — PROYECTO BILINGUE

TRANSCRIPTION — TRANSCRIPCION

Complete the following report along with the completed transcription. (See pp. 107-108).

Prepare la siguiente transcripción y termine los informes adjuntos (Vea pág. 107-108).

NAME — NOMBRE: _____

ADDRESS — DIRECCION:_____

SITUATION — SITUACION: _____

This 62 year-old man was first noticed by his wife kneeling on the kitchen floor clutching his chest and struggling for breath. He was taken to the hospital by ambulance. Initial evaluation was not conclusive. He was seen in consultation and with the aid of special tests, a diagnosis of a blood clot in the lung was made. Treatment was successful and he was discharged 13 days later.

A este señor de 62 años de edad lo encontró su esposa en la cocina arrodillado, apretándose el pecho y forcejeando por respirar. Fue llevado en ambulancia al hospital. La evaluación inicial no fue definitiva. Lo observaron varios médicos consultantes y, con la ayuda de algunos exámenes, se diagnosticó que tenía un coágulo en el pulmón. El tratamiento resultó efectivo y fue dado de alta a los 13 días.

SEQUENCE OF REPORTS   —   ORDEN DE LOS INFORMES:

A—1

History and Physical Exam
Historia y examen físico

Completed _____

Terminado _____

A—2

X-ray Report
Informe radiológico

Completed _____

Terminado _____

A—3

X-ray Report (lung scan)
Informe radiológico
del pulmón
Completed _____

Terminado _____

A—4

Consultants' Report
Informe de los consultantes

Completed _____

Terminado _____

A—5

Clinical Resumé
Resumen clínico

Completed _____

Terminado _____

EXERCISES — EJERCICIOS

(Students learning Spanish — Estudiantes de español)

A. Rewrite the following sentences and replace the underlined nouns with direct object pronouns.

1. El cirujano hace la operación. ....

2. Las enfermeras buscan las medicinas. ....

3. Los pacientes toman los remedios. ....

4. El jefe envía la receta. ....

5. Evito el contagio. ....

B. Rewrite the following sentences and replace the underlined words with direct and indirect object pronouns.

e.g. Ella trae la medicina para mi   —Ella me la trae.

   El busca un cuadro para su novia — Se lo busca. El se lo busca.

1. El doctor escribe la receta para el paciente.

2. La enfermera trae las pastillas para nosotros. ....

3. Le estoy leyendo un libro al enfermo. ....

4. Vamos a comprar los ungüentos para el hospital. ....

5. La empleada pone una vacuna al pescador. ....

C. Translate into Spanish.

1. His son came to him. ....   3. He is coming with me. ....

2. This book is for me. ....   4. Do you know her? ....

D. Write a short composition dealing with communicable diseases.

....

....

....

E. Answer in Spanish.

1. ¿Por qué son peligrosas las enfermedades venéreas? ....

2. ¿Cómo se puede evitar el contagio con una persona enferma? ....

   ....

3. ¿Cómo trata el hospital las enfermedades contagiosas? ....

   ....

4. ¿Por qué es importante la microbiología? ....

5. ¿Para qué sirven las vacunas? ....

EJERCICIOS — EXERCISES

(Estudiantes de inglés — Students learning English)

A. Traduzca las siguientes oraciones al inglés.

1. El paciente se toma la medicina. Se la toma. ....

2. Ella nos lee el libro. Nos lo lee. ....

3. Vamos donde el doctor y él nos examina. ....

4. La vimos en el hospital. ....

5. Es una enfermedad muy contagiosa. ....

B. Conteste en inglés.

1. What is the best medicine for tuberculosis? ....

2. Why is syphilis dangerous? ....

3. How do you treat a contagious disease? ....

4. Why is microbiology so important? ....

5. Why are antibiotics necessary? ....

C. Escriba una composición corta sobre enfermedades contagiosas.

....

....

D. Escriba seis oraciones con formas de verbos defectivos.

1. ....   4. ....

2. ....   5. ....

3. ....   6. ....

E. Escriba un diálogo corto relacionado con una visita al doctor.
Tenga en cuenta las siguientes expresiones:

It's better to take antibiotics   — es mejor tomar antibióticos.

Is there a preventive method?   — ¿hay un método preventivo?

What symptoms do you have?   — ¿qué síntomas tiene?

How long have you been feeling better?   — ¿cuánto tiempo hace que usted se siente mejor?

Yes, you have a contagious disease.   — sí, usted tiene una enfermedad contagiosa.

It's in the advanced stage.   — está en estado avanzado.

....

....

....

....

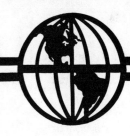

CARING FOR THE BED PATIENT
EL CUIDADO DEL PACIENTE EN CAMA

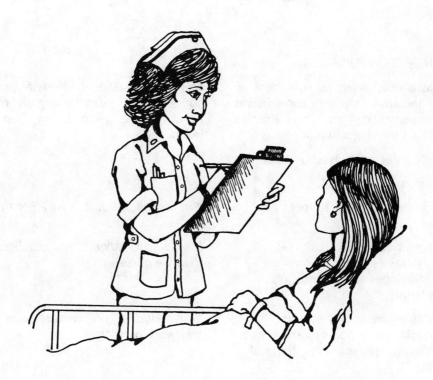

VOCABULARY — VOCABULARIO

A. Medical — Médico

aislamiento	— isolation	cuidado de la enfermera	— nursing care
apatía	— apathy	deseos	— wants
apetito	— appetite	medios, recursos de laboratorio	— laboratory facilities
bulla innecesaria, ruido innecesario	— noisy fuss, unnecessary noise		
baño	— bath	programa diario	— daily schedule
clínica de reposo	— nursing home	remedio	— remedy, medicine
consejo médico	— doctor's or medical advice	siesta	— nap
		veterinario	— veterinarian

B. General

acomodar	— to accommodate	insistir	— to insist
alarmar	— to alarm	libertad	— freedom
antes	— before	llevar	— to carry, take
compartir	— to share	ocupado	— busy
después	— after	pesado	— heavy
en cambio	— on the other hand	posible	— possible
enrojecer	— to redden	salir	— to leave
exagerar	— to overdo, exaggerate	terminar	— to finish
imponer a la fuerza	— to enforce	traer	— to bring
información	— information	ver	— to see

CONVERSATION — CONVERSACION

A. Mercedes Castañeda, quien es enfermera en un asilo para ancianos y que está aprendiendo inglés, se encuentra con su amiga Rosalva Peña, maestra de escuela primaria.

Mercedes Castañeda, who is a nurse in a nursing home and is learning English met her friend Rosalva Peña, who is an Elementary school teacher.

Rosalva — Hola, Mercedes, ¿cómo estás?

Mercedes — Bien, gracias, ¿y tú?

Rosalva — No tan bien como tú, pero ahí vamos.

Not as well as you but we'll get there.

Mercedes — Miren quien habla. Uds. las maestras están en mejores condiciones que nosotras las enfermeras.

Look who is talking. You teachers are better off than we nurses.

Rosalva — Estás bromeando. Nosotras trabajamos 24 horas mientras que Uds. trabajan sólo ocho horas al día.

You're kidding. We work 24 hours a day while you work only eight.

Mercedes — Pero tu programa no es tan pesado como el nuestro.

But your schedule is not as heavy as ours.

Rosalva — ¿Cuál es tu programa diario?

What's your daily schedule?

Mercedes — Si me permites te diré cuál es mi programa con un solo paciente.

If you'll allow me I'll tell you what my schedule is with just one patient.

Rosalva — Dímelo en inglés.

Tell me in English.

Mercedes — When I get to the hospital the nurse on shift gives me all the information concerning the patient.
When he wakes up, I brush his teeth and take him to the bathroom.
Then I give him a bath, comb his hair and dress him.

1. *Cuando llego al hospital la enfermera en turno me da toda la información acerca del paciente.*

2. *Cuando se despierta le lavo la boca y lo llevo al baño.*

3. *Luego le doy un baño, lo peino y lo visto.*

Then I bring him his food.
I try to keep him happy all day,
and I make him take a nap.
And before I leave I give all the
information to the nurse who
comes to take my place.

4. *Después le traigo sus alimentos.*

5. *Procuro que esté contento todo el día y que duerma una siesta.*
6. *Y antes de irme le doy toda la información a la enfermera que llega a reemplazarme.*

Rosalva — Tienes razón, tu trabajo es más pesado que el nuestro.

GRAMMATICAL HINTS — APUNTES GRAMATICALES

A. Comparisons in Spanish

1. Comparisons of equality

In comparing adjectives and adverbs, **as ... as** is expressed by **tan ... como**:
El es **tan** inteligente **como** su hermana — He is **as** intelligent **as** his sister.
Viene **tan** rápido **como** puede — He comes **as** fast **as** he can.

In comparing nouns, **as** much (many) ... **as,** is expressed by **tanto** (os), **tanta** (as) ... **como**:
No muestro **tanta** iniciativa **como** tú — I don't show **as** much iniciative **as** you (do).
Ella escribe **tantas** cartas **como** su amiga — She writes **as** many letters **as** her friend (does).

2. Comparisons of inequality
   a) The comparison of inequality is regularly formed by placing **más** o **menos** before the positive form of adjectives and adverbs. The word **than** is usually expressed by **que**.
   El niño está **más** enfermo **que** el adulto — The child is sicker than the adult.
   El farmacéutico es **menos** cuidadoso **que** su compañero — The pharmacist is less careful than his companion.
   b) Before cardinal numbers **than** is expressed by **de**.
   El estará más **de** dos semanas en el hospital.
   c) The superlative is formed by placing the definite article before the comparative form. **De** renders English **in**.
   El es **el** enfermo más paciente **de** todo el hospital (in the whole hospital).
   d) There are four adjectives and four adverbs which are compared irregularly.

Adjectives		Adverbs	
bueno	— mejor (más bueno)	bien	— mejor
malo	— peor (más malo)	mal	— peor
grande	— mayor (más grande)	mucho	— más
pequeño	— menor (más pequeño)	poco	— menos

El policía es **mejor** que el detective.

B. Comparación de adjetivos en inglés

1. La comparación de igualdad entre dos objetos o personas se forma poniendo **as** antes y después del adjetivo.
e.g. Mary is **as** intelligent **as** her sister.

2. En la comparación de superioridad los adjetivos tienen tres grados de comparación: en la forma positiva, por ejemplo se dice **big** (grande), en la comparativa **bigger** (más grande) y en la superlativa **biggest** (el o la más grande, el o la mayor). Es necesario decir luego que hay dos formas de hacer esta clase de comparación:

a) Agregando los sufijos **er** y **est** a los adjetivos de una sola sílaba: **er** para los comparativos y **est** para los superlativos.

e.g. sweet, sweeter, sweetest — dulce, más dulce, el más dulce.

b) Usando **more** and **most** con los adjetivos de más de dos sílabas.

e.g. He is **more** intelligent **than** his brother — El es más inteligente que su hermano

(nótese que **que** se traduce **than**).

3. Las comparaciones siguientes son irregulares:

Positivo	Comparativo	Superlativo
good	better	best
bad, ill	worse	worst
much	more	most
many	more	most
little	less	least
old	older, elder	oldest, eldest
far	farther, further	farthest, furthest

4. En la comparación de inferioridad se usa **less** y **least.**

e.g. The patient is **less** intelligent **than** his roommate —

El paciente es menos inteligente que su compañero de cuarto.

He is the **least** intelligent of them all — El es el menos inteligente de todos.

C. Los adverbios se comparan tal como los adjetivos:

e.g. quickly, more quickly, most quickly — rápido, más rápido, (lo) más rápido.

soon, sooner, soonest — pronto, más pronto, (lo) más pronto.

often, less often, least often — a menudo, menos a menudo, (lo) menos a menudo.

CONVERSATION — CONVERSACION (Cont.)

B. The Rentería's child woke up very sick, and his parents called Dr. Richardson. He arrived at the house. After he examined the child he gave these instructions to the parents. A friend of the family did the translating.

El niño de los Rentería amaneció muy enfermo y sus padres llamaron al Dr. Richardson. El llegó a la casa, y después de examinarlo les dió estas instrucciones a los padres. Una amiga de la familia hizo la traducción.

1. Don't make any unnecessary fuss.

No le hagan bulla innecesaria.

2. Don't force him to eat.

No lo obliguen a comer.

3. Give him the medicine on time.

Dénle la medicina a tiempo.

4. Don't leave him by himself.

No lo dejen en aislamiento.

5. Check his temperature regularly.

Tómenle regularmente la temperatura.

6. Try to keep him happy.

Traten de mantenerlo contento.

7. If there are any complication's be sure to call me again.

Si hay alguna complicación, llámenme de nuevo.

GRAMMATICAL HINTS — APUNTES GRAMATICALES (Cont.)

D. El futuro en español

1. The future tense in Spanish is formed by adding the following endings to the infinitive form of all verbs.

Hablar**é**	— I will speak
ás	you (fam. sing.) will speak
á	he, she, you (for. sing.) will speak
emos	we will speak
án	they, you (plu.) will speak

2. There are a few irregular verbs in the future. Some of them are:

tener	— tendré	poder	— podré
hacer	— haré	salir	— saldré
decir	— diré	venir	— vendré
poner	— pondré	querer	— querré
saber	— sabré		

E. El futuro en inglés

1. El futuro se forma poniendo el verbo imperfecto **will** antes del verbo en infinitivo.
e.g. I will do the work — Haré el trabajo.

2. Se usa también la contracción para indicar el futuro.
e.g. We'll be back someday — volveremos algún día.

3. Shall también se usa para indicar el futuro pero raras veces. Este verbo imperfecto se usa más bien en preguntas, especialmente cuando nos dirigimos a una persona y le preguntamos lo que ella quiere que hagamos.
e.g. Shall we close the door? — ¿cerramos la puerta?
     Shall we talk?   — ¿hablamos?

4. Otra forma de expresar el futuro es usando **to be going to.**
e.g. The surgeon is going to operate today — el cirujano va a operar hoy.

CONVERSATION — CONVERSACION (Cont.)

C. Mary Lamb was assigned to give a lecture about the importance of nursing homes. Her lecture began this way...

A Mary Lamb le asignaron la tarea de dar una conferencia acerca de la importancia de las clínicas de reposo. Ella comenzó su disertación de la siguiente manera...

In recent years, nursing homes have had a considerable increase in patients. As with hospitals, nursing homes offer good services in varying ways. Even though they do not have lab facilities or a resident doctor in a nursing home, patients receive first class service and care. The main service offered in these nursing homes of course, that of serving patients, especially the very old.

En los últimos años las clínicas de reposo han tenido un aumento considerable en el número de pacientes. Tal como los hospitales, ofrecen un buen servicio en distintos aspectos. Aunque no tienen recursos de laboratorio y no hay un doctor residente en la clínica, las atenciones hacia el paciente son de primera clase. El servicio principal que ofrecen estas clínicas de reposo es, desde luego, prestarle un servicio al paciente, especialmente a los ancianos.

ADDITIONAL INFORMATION — INFORMACION ADICIONAL

1. Athletic terms — Términos atléticos

aficionado (amatero)	— amateur	evento	— event
árbitro	— referee, umpire	ganar, ganador	— to win, winner
atleta	— athlete	juego, partido	— game, match
campeón	— champion	juegos olímpicos	— Olympic games
campo, cancha	— field, court	juez	— judge
capitán	— captain	jugada	— play
competencia, torneo	— competition, tournament	jugador	— player
competidor	— competitor	perder, perdedor	— to lose, loser
copa	— cup	profesional	— professional
entrenador (coach)	— coach, trainer	tantos, puntos (score)	— score, points
estadio	— stadium		

2. Spanish last names   Apellidos ingleses

Azuela	Ospina	Abbott	Black
Bueno	Porras	Adams	Bolden
Carrasco	Restrepo	Alexander	Bowman
Durán	Rivera	Baker	Boyd
Duque	Suárez	Bell	Brown
Espinoza	Valencia	Benson	
Juárez	Verdugo		
Liévano	Villamil		

3. Useful expressions — Expresiones útiles

El paciente puede recibir visitas	— The patient can receive visitors.
Tome este remedio cuando sienta el dolor	— Take this remedy whenever you feel pain.
Niños menores de catorce años no pueden visitar	— Children under 14 can't visit.
No tome ninguna medicina casera	— Do not take any home remedy.
¿Estoy mejor o peor?	— Am I better or worse?
¿Tiene escalofríos?	— Do you have chills?
Este es un hospital general	— This is a general hospital.
¿Qué te pasa?	— What's the matter with you?
Tiene que tomarse la medicina	— You have to take your medicine.
Voy a hacerle la cama	— I am going to make your bed.
Con un compañero de cuarto	— With a roommate.

4. Idiomatic expressions — Expresiones idiomáticas

A grandes rasgos	— Briefly, without going into detail	Largos años	— A long time
		Llamar la atención	— To call or attract attention to
Comoquiera que sea	— In any case		
Cortar al prójimo	— Criticize one's neighbor	Mucho ruido y pocas nueces	— Much ado about nothing
Cuatro letras	— A few lines	Ni para remedio	— Not for love or money
En el fondo	— By nature, at bottom, at heart		
		Saber lo que es bueno	— To know what one is missing
Forjarse o hacerse ilusiones	— To build castles in the air	Sin novedad	— As usual

5. Some more medical terms — Más términos médicos

aguja	— needle	gasa	— gauze
almohadilla	— cushion	guantes de gaucho o	
antídotos para		de goma	— rubber gloves
envenenamientos	— antidotes for poison	hemostato	— hemostat
aparatos ortopédicos	— orthopedic braces,	hisopo	— cotton swab
	supports, etc.	laminilla de vidrio	— glass slide
audiómetro	— audiometer	laringoscopio	— laryngoscope
bata de operaciones	— operating gown	martillo de percusión	— percussion hammer
bolsa de hielo	— ice bag	mascarilla	— mask
boquilla	— mouthpiece	mesa de operaciones	— operating table
botiquín	— first-aid kit	microscopio	— microscope
caja de Petri	— Petri dish	muletas	— crutches
caucho, goma	— rubber	oftalmoscopio	— ophtalmoscope
colcha	— cover	pera de goma	— rubber bulb
colchón	— mattress	pinzas, tenazas	— forceps
cuentagotas	— medicine dropper	pulmón de hierro	— iron lung
electrocardiograma	— electrocardiogram	silla de operaciones	— operating chair
electroencefalograma	— electroencephalogram	sulfato de calcio	— calcium sulfate
enema	— enema	venda de goma	— rubber bandage
espejuelos, gafas,			
lentes	— eyeglasses		

6. More medical supplies — Más provisiones médicas

báscula	— scale	palangana lavatorio	— washbasin
bisturí, escapelo,		paños esterilizados	— sterile cloths
lanceta	— scalpel, lancet	pisalengua	— tongue depressor
bomba estomacal	— stomach pump	rayos X	— X rays
braguero	— truss, brace	sábanas	— sheets
camilla	— stretcher	sonda	— sound, probe
diapasón	— tuning fork	supositorio	— suppository
estetoscopio	— stethoscope	sutura, suturar	— suture, to suture
estilete	— stylet, probe	tablilla	— splint
faja abdominal	— swathing bandage	tapón	— surgical tampon
imperdible, seguro	— safety pin	termómetro	— thermometer
jeringuilla	— syringe	tijeras	— scissors
lavamanos	— wash stand	tubo de ensayo	— test-tube

BILINGUAL PROJECT — PROYECTO BILINGUE

TRANSCRIPTION — TRANSCRIPCION

Complete the following report along with the completed transcription. (See pp. 107-108).

Prepare la siguiente transcripción y termine los informes adjuntos.(Vea pág. 107-108).

NAME — NOMBRE: _____

ADDRESS — DIRECCION: _____

SITUATION — SITUACION:

This 23 year-old woman was admitted to the hospital because of severe abdominal pain and vaginal bleeding. After an initial evaluation and an X-ray study, she was taken to surgery where examination and surgical exploration revealed an ectopic pregnancy, which was removed. The pathology report confirmed the diagnosis. She convalesced well and was discharged home one week after admission.

Esta mujer de 23 años de edad fue admitida al hospital por tener dolores agudos en el abdomen y un flujo de sangre por la vagina. Después de una evaluación inicial y un estudio radiográfico, fue llevada a la cirugía donde se le hizo un examen y una exploración quirúrgica que revelaron tener un embarazo ectópico, el cual fue extraído. El informe patológico confirmó el diagnóstico. Convaleció bien y fue dada de alta una semana después de su admisión.

SEQUENCE OF REPORTS   —   ORDEN DE LOS INFORMES:

A—1

History and Physical Exam
Historia y examen físico

Completed _____

Terminado _____

A—2

X-ray Report
Informe radiológico

Completed _____

Terminado _____

A—3

Operative Record
Informe quirúrgico

Completed _____

Terminado _____

A—4

Pathology Report
Informe patológico

Completed _____

Terminado _____

A—5

Clinical Resumé
Resumen clínico

Completed _____

Terminado _____

EXERCISES — EJERCICIOS

(Students learning Spanish — Estudiantes de español)

A. Fill in the blank in each of the following sentences by selecting the appropriate form in parentheses.

1. Ella es _____ buena como su prima. (tanto, tan, tanta)

2. El paciente es _____ amable como el doctor. (tanta, tan, tanto)

3. Leo la carta. _____ leo. (lo, la, las)

4. Este es _____ hospital. (nuestro, nuestra, nuestros)

5. El maneja tan rápido _____ la enfermera. (tantos, cual, como)

B. Translate the underlined words.

1. Nuestro hospital tiene **as many** camas **as** el Hospital General. . . . .

2. La sala de maternidad es **as** grande **as** la farmacia. . . . .

3. Es **better** no discutir con los pacientes. . . . .

4. Juan tiene **more than** cinco medicamentos que tomar. . . . .

5. El técnico tiene **as many** pacientes **as** el médico. . . . .

C. Write four sentences with idiomatic expressions.

1. . . . .   3. . . . .

2. . . . .   4. . . . .

D. Change the following sentences from present to future.

1. El paciente come la comida. . . . .

2. Las enfermeras bañan al inválido. . . . .

3. Luis y María se quieren mucho. . . . .

4. Yo hablo español e inglés. . . . .

5. Los gérmenes son peligrosos. . . . .

E. Answer in complete Spanish.

1. ¿Tiene Ud. mareo? . . . .

2. ¿Cómo cuida Ud. a un paciente? . . . .

3. ¿Por qué está Ud. contento? . . . .

4. Mencione algunas enfermedades contagiosas. . . . .

5. ¿Qué preparativos se hacen para un paciente que llega al hospital? . . . .

. . . .

F. Write a letter to a hospital asking for information about the results of laboratory tests performed on a patient ten days previously.

EJERCICIOS — EXERCISES

(Estudiantes de inglés — Students learning English)

A. Haga una comparación con los adjetivos en paréntesis.

1. Gary is _____ (tall) _____ his friend.

2. The weather is _____ (hot) _____ last week.

3. Peter is _____ (popular) _____ Charles.

4. To read English is much _____ (easy) _____ to speak it.

5. Mary's work this quarter is _____ (bad) _____ it was last quarter.

B. Tradúzcanse las siguientes oraciones.

1. Nuestro hospital tiene tantas camas como el Hospital General. ....

2. La sala de maternidad es tan grande como la farmacia. ....

3. El técnico tiene menos pacientes que el doctor. ....

4. Esa es la mejor clínica de la ciudad. ....

5. El enfermo es mejor que el enfermero. ....

C. Llene el espacio vacío con la forma adverbial del adjetivo dado entre paréntesis, recordando que para formar un adverbio se añade ly al final de la mayoría de los adjetivos.

1. You pronounce each word very _____ (distinct).

2. The nurse works more _____ (careful) than anybody else.

3. The doctor comes as _____ (frequent) as the nurse.

4. The price of this car has risen _____ (rapid) over the past several months.

5. This patient is improving _____ (gradual).

D. Cambie las oraciones siguientes del presente al futuro.

1. The patient eats his food. ....

2. The nurses take care of the patient. ....

3. I speak English and French. ....

4. The hospital has many beds. ....

5. The sick man feels better. ....

E. Conteste las siguientes preguntas en inglés.

1. ¿Qué piensa hacer Ud. mañana? ....

2. ¿Cómo debe cuidarse a un paciente? ....

3. ¿Tiene Ud. algún amigo que esté enfermo? ¿Cuál es su problema? ....

4. ¿Qué profesión le gustaría escoger? ....

5. ¿Por qué es importante la medicina? ....

F. Escriba una carta a un hospital pidiendo información acerca de los resultados de las pruebas de laboratorio hechas a un paciente hace diez días.

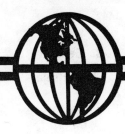

MATERNITY
MATERNIDAD

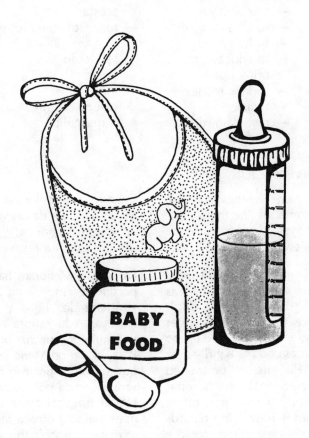

VOCABULARY — VOCABULARIO

A. Medical — Médico

aborto	— abortion, miscarriage
alumbramiento, parto	— birth, delivery
anticonceptivo	— contraceptive
atención prenatal	— prenatal care
bebé, criatura	— baby
bolsa de agua, bolsa amniótica	— amnion, amniotic sack, bag of waters
concepción	— conception
dolores de parto	— labor pains
embarazo, estado de gestación	— pregnancy
encinta, embarazada	— pregnant

factor Rh	— Rh factor
feto	— fetus
ginecólogo	— gynecologist
obstetra	— obstetrician
óvulo	— ovum
parir, alumbrar, dar a luz	— to give birth (to), deliver
partera	— midwife
paternidad responsable	— planned parenthood
planificación familiar	— family planning
regla, menstruación	— menstrual period
sala de maternidad	— maternity ward

B. General

aconsejar	— to advise, give advice	leer	— to read
ayudar	— to help	llevar	— to take, carry
biberón	— nursing bottle	membrana	— membrane
consejo	— advice	método	— method
construir	— to build	nacer	— to be born
contar con	— to count on	ofrecer	— to offer
cuidar a	— to take care of	prestar	— to lend
darse prisa	— to hurry	reconstruir, remodelar	— to reconstruct, rebuild, remodel
educar	— to educate, raise, bring up	resultado	— result
faltarle a uno dinero	— to lack money	tetera	— nipple on a baby bottle
hembra	— female	varón, varonil, masculino	— male, masculine
leche en polvo	— dry or powdered milk		

CONVERSATION — CONVERSACION

A. When the ambulance came to the home of the Mendoza family, one of the neighbors inquired about Mrs. Mendoza and a friend of the family gave the following answer.

Mrs. Mendoza has to go to the hospital because she began to have labor pains. She has two children and now she is expecting a third. Mrs. Mendoza would like to have a daughter because the other two are boys. According to Mr. Mendoza, a boy is just as good as a girl, so he doesn't worry about that. His wife will be treated by the best doctors in the hospital. The hospital has a very good maternity ward that offers excellent service. The ward is now being remodeled and they plan to build new offices for the doctors. The main entrance is now by way of the emergency ward. When the construction work is terminated, this hospital will be one of the best in the community.

Cuando la ambulancia vino al hogar de la familia Mendoza, una de las vecinas preguntó acerca de la señora Mendoza, y una amiga de la familia dio la siguiente respuesta.

La señora Mendoza ha tenido que ir al hospital porque le empezaron los dolores del parto. Ella ya tiene dos hijos y ahora está esperando el tercero. A la señora Mendoza le gustaría tener una niña porque sus otros dos hijos son varones. Para el señor Mendoza lo mismo es una niña que un niño, por eso no se preocupa. Su esposa será atendida por los mejores médicos del hospital. El hospital tiene un buen departamento de maternidad y ofrece muy buena atención. Ahora lo están remodelando y piensan construir nuevas oficinas para los doctores. La entrada principal está ahora por la sala de emergencia. Cuando se termine la nueva construcción este hospital será uno de los mejores de la comunidad.

GRAMMATICAL HINTS — APUNTES GRAMATICALES

A. Para y por

The prepositions **para** and **por** are not interchangeable even though they frequently mean **for** in English. Generally speaking **para** indicates:

1. Direction toward a destination.
El doctor salió **para** Argentina.

2. Intention, purpose, goal.
Lupe estudia **para** enfermera. **(to become)**

3. For whom something is intended.
Construyeron oficinas nuevas **para** los doctores.

4. The special use or purpose of an object.
Quiere un cepillo **para** el pelo.

Por, on the other hand, expresses:

1. Approximate time.
Tiene una cita **por** la mañana.

2. Passing through, along or by a place or area.
La entrada principal es ahora **por** la sala de emergencia.

3. The agent by whom an action is performed.
Su esposa quiere ser atendida **por** los mejores doctores.

4. Cause or reason why something is done.
Lo hizo **por** amor a su hijo.

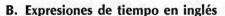

B. Expresiones de tiempo en inglés

Las expresiones de tiempo definido se ponen al final de la oración precedidas por las de lugar.
e.g. It's cold here **today** — **hace** frío hoy.
    It's hot in the desert **all the time** — **hace** mucho calor en el desierto todo el tiempo.
    It's warm in the summer — hace calor en el verano.
    I usually get up at 7 o'clock — por lo general me levanto a las siete.

CONVERSATION — CONVERSACION (Cont.)

B. Mrs. Ernestina Ortiz was taken to the hospital because she is about ready to have her baby. Mrs. Mara Cardozo, the nurse, does the necessary translating.

La señora Ernestina Ortiz fue llevada al hospital porque está cerca de dar a luz. La señora Mara Cardozo, la enfermera, hace la traducción necesaria.

Doctor	— What time did your labor pains begin, Mrs. Ortiz?	*¿A qué hora le empezaron los dolores, Sra. Ortiz?*
Mara	— ¿A qué hora le empezaron los dolores, Sra. Ortiz?	
Ernestina	— Esta mañana cerca de las nueve.	*This morning about nine.*
Mara	— This morning about nine.	
Doctor	— How many minutes apart?	*¿Con cuánta frecuencia?*
Mara	— ¿Con cuánta frecuencia?	
Ernestina	— Cada cinco minutos.	*Every five minutes.*
Mara	— Every five minutes.	
Doctor	— Is this your first baby?	*¿Es éste su primer hijo?*
Mara	— ¿Es éste su primer hijo?	
Ernestina	— Sí, el primero.	*Yes, the first.*
Mara	— Yes, the first.	
Doctor	— Have you had any other pregnancies?	*¿Ha tenido algunos otros embarazos?*
Mara	— ¿Ha tenido algunos otros embarazos?	

Ernestina	— Sí, hace dos años.		*Yes, two years ago.*
Mara	— Yes, two years ago.		

Doctor	— Did you have a miscarriage?		*¿tuvo un aborto?*
Mara	— ¿Tuvo un aborto?		
Ernestina	— Sí.		
Mara	— Yes.		

Doctor	— Is your blood type Rh positive or negative?		*¿Es su tipo de sangre Rh positiva o negativa?*
Mara	— ¿Es su tipo de sangre Rh positiva o negativa?		
Ernestina	— No sé. Tal vez la oficina tenga esa información en mi registro médico.		*I don't know. Maybe the office has that information in my medical record.*
Mara	— Perhaps we can get that information in the medical record.		
Doctor	— Do you know if your bag of waters has broken?		*¿Sabe si su bolsa de agua ya se reventó?*
Mara	— ¿Sabe si su bolsa de agua ya se reventó?		
Ernestina	— Creo que no.		*I don't think so.*
Mara	— She doesn't think so.		
Doctor	— Thank you very much, Mrs. Ortiz. This is all the information we need.		*Mil gracias señora Ortiz. Esta es toda la información que necesitamos.*
Mara	— Gracias, señora Ortiz. Esta es toda la información que necesitamos.		

GRAMMATICAL HINTS — APUNTES GRAMATICALES

C. The conditional in Spanish

The conditional, as the name implies, is a mood that expresses an action dependent on a condition. It is formed by adding a group of special endings to the same stem that we used for the future tense in the previous lesson.

yo estar**ía**

tú estar**ías**

él
ella estar**ía**
Ud.

nosotros
nosotras estar**íamos**

} en la sala de maternidad.

ellos
ellas estar**ían**
Uds.

These endings are regular whether they are attached to a regular stem or to an irregular one.

D. Oraciones condicionales en inglés

Una oración condicional es aquélla que contiene dos cláusulas, una dependiente con **if** (si) y la cláusula principal como respuesta a la condición.

e.g. If the doctor comes, he will see the patient — Si viene el doctor verá al paciente.

Las oraciones condicionales son de tres formas: 1) Futuro de posibilidad. 2)Presente irreal. 3) Pasado irreal.

1. El futuro de posibilidad es una condición en la cual se usa el tiempo presente en la cláusula **if** y el futuro en la respuesta.
e.g. If the nurse has time, she will work today — si la enfermera tiene tiempo trabajará hoy.

2. El presente irreal es una condición en la cual se usa el tiempo pasado en la cláusula **if** y **would** (**could** o **might**) como auxiliar del verbo en la segunda cláusula. Esta es la condición contraria a los hechos que se usa en castellano con el imperfecto del subjuntivo en la cláusula **si** (if) y el condicional en la cláusula principal.
e.g. If I had money, I would go to England — si tuviera dinero iría a Inglaterra (esto quiere decir que en efecto **no tengo** dinero ahora).
If John knew how to swim, he would do it every day — Si Juan supiera nadar lo haría todos los días.
If the doctor **were** here, he would help us — si el doctor estuviera aquí nos ayudaría (nótese la forma **were**).

3. El pasado irreal es una condición que indica una situación hipotética que es irreal y contraria a los hechos. (Vea pág. 155).
e.g. If he had studied, he would have passed his examinations —
si hubiera estudiado habría aprobado los exámenes (quiere decir que **no** estudio).

4. La oración hipotética del futuro se refiere a una posibilidad futura pero en cierto grado remota.
e.g. If he arrived (were to arrive) on time tomorrow, we could conclude the deal —
si él llegara a tiempo mañana, podríamos concluir el trato.

E. Augmentatives and diminutives in Spanish

1. The most common augmentative suffixes are **ón, azo, ote,** and **acho,** which imply large size, ugliness, awkwardness or excess.
e.g. mujer — mujerona   pobre — pobretón
señor — señorón

2. The diminutive suffixes are much more common than the augmentative ones, and they are important for understanding the correct shades of meaning implied. The most common ones are **ito, cito, ecito; illo, cillo, ecillo; uelo; uco;** and **ucho.** The endings **ito, illo** with their longer forms, and **uelo,** denote smallness of size, endearment, and affection.
They are used with nouns and adjectives.
e.g. pájaro — pajarito   solo — solito
pueblo — pueblecito   viejo — viejecito

ADDITIONAL INFORMATION — INFORMACION ADICIONAL

1. More Vocabulary — Más vocabulario

alumbramiento múltiple	— multiple birth	pesario intrauterino	— pessary, intrauterine (contraceptive) device, IUD
alumbramiento (parto) prematuro	— premature birth		
alumbramiento sencillo	— single birth	peso al nacer	— weight at birth
antojo	— craving during pregnancy	placenta	— placenta
		presentación de cabeza	— head presentation
		presentación de nalgas	— breech presentation
ansias matutinas	— morning sickness	prueba de embarazo	— pregnancy test
dar el pecho (la teta)	— to breast-feed	relaciones sexuales	— sexual relations
defectos de nacimiento	— birth defects	sala de parto	— delivery room
examen de orina, urinálisis	— urinalysis	se rompió la bolsa de agua	— the bag of waters has broken
embrión	— embryo	sietemesino	— seven-month baby
examen de sangre	— blood test	sobreparto, post partum	— period of time immediately after birth
lactante	— lactating		
madres primerizas	— new mothers		
mellizos	— twins	tener el pelo castaño	— to have dark hair
operación cesárea	— Caesarian operation or section	tener el pelo rubio	— to have light colored hair (not necessarily blond)
peligro de aborto	— danger of miscarriage	vómitos persistentes	— persistent vomiting

2. Commands — Mandatos

descanse	— rest	no respire tan profundo	— don't breathe so deep
empuje	— push		
levante la cabeza	— raise your head	pare	— stop
mantenga la respiración y luego empuje	— hold your breath and then push	respire profundamente	— take a deep breath

3. More commands — Más mandatos

No la dejemos aquí	— Let's not leave her (it) here.	Que llueva	— Let it rain.
No vayamos al hospital	— Let's not go to the hospital.	Que venga el paciente	— Let the patient come.
		Vámonos	— Let's go.
Que lo haga el doctor	— Let the doctor do it.	Vamos a casa	— Let's go home.

4. Useful Expressions — Expresiones útiles

No hay complicaciones	— There are no complications.
Acuéstese aquí, por favor	— Please lie down here.
Le voy a tomar la temperatura	— I'm going to take your temperature.
Llámeme por favor si tiene preguntas	— Please call me if you have any questions
Usted está en buenas manos	— You are in good hands.
¿Necesita ir al baño?	— Do you have to go to the bathroom?
Es la hora de su baño	— It's time for your bath.
Toque el timbre una vez	— Ring the bell once.
¿Puede haber complicaciones con la píldora?	— Can there be complications from the pill?

¿Quién es su doctor?   — Who is your doctor?
¿Para qué sirven los anticonceptivos?   — What are contraceptives good for?
¿Qué son los profilácticos?   — What are prophylactics?
¿Está embarazada?   — Are you pregnant?
¿Cuál es su tipo sanguíneo?   — What is your blood type?

5. Idioms — Modismos

en primer lugar   — in the first place   muy pronto   — very soon
guardar cama   — to stay in bed   nada del otro mundo   — (It's) nothing
guardar silencio   — to keep silent or   unusual
                      quiet   tener inconveniente   — to have an
horas de consulta   — office hours   objection, a reason
horas de visita   — visiting hours   for not doing
mil cosas   — many things   something

6. Spanish Last Names   Apellidos ingleses

Beltrán   Rojas   Bold   Bradley
Chávez   Tovar   Bradford   Brady
Cortés   Brett
Díaz   Broods
Martín   Buchanan
Osorio   Burns
Pereda   Burt
Rendón   Butler
                                           Campbell
                                           Carlson

breast / mama
umbilical cord / cordón umbilical
placenta / placenta
amniotic sac / bolsa amniótica
amniotic fluid / líquido amniótico
fetus / feto
uterus / útero
rectum / intestino recto
cervix / cuello uterino
cervical canal / canal cervical
urethra / uretra
vagina / vagina

BILINGUAL PROJECT — PROYECTO BILINGUE

TRANSCRIPTION — TRANSCRIPCION

Complete the following report along with the completed transcription. (See pp. 107-108).

Prepare la siguiente transcripción y termine los informes adjuntos. (Vea pág. 107-108).

NAME — NOMBRE: _____

ADDRESS — DIRECCION: _____

SITUATION — SITUACION:

This 29 year-old female suffering from severe abdominal cramps, nausea, and vomiting was rushed to the medical center emergency room on May 16, 19__. Here she was examined and admitted to the hospital with a tentative diagnosis of appendicitis. Blood test were done and X-rays taken, then she was taken to surgery. An acutely inflamed appendix was removed and her convalescence was uneventful. She was discharged one week after admission.

Esta mujer de 29 años de edad sufría de calambres abdominales agudos, náuseas y vómitos y fue traída de emergencia al hospital el 16 de mayo de 19__. Aquí fue examinada y admitida al hospital con un diagnóstico tentativo de apendicitis. Se le estudió la sangre y se le tomaron radiografías, y luego fue llevada a la cirugía. Un apéndice muy inflamado se le sacó y su convalescencia fue sin contratiempo alguno. Se le dio de alta una semana después de ser admitida.

SEQUENCE OF REPORTS   —   ORDEN DE LOS INFORMES:

A—1

History and Physical Exam
Historia y examen físico
Completed
Terminado _____

A—2

X-ray Report
Informe radiológico
Completed
Terminado _____

A—3

Operative Record
registro quirúrgico
Completed
Terminado _____

A—4

Pathology Report
Informe patológico
Completed
Terminado _____

A—5

Clinical Resumé
Resumen clínico
Completed
Terminado _____

EXERCISES — EJERCICIOS

(Students learning Spanish — Estudiantes de Español

A. Fill in the blanks with para or por.

1. El sale _____ México y va _____ El Paso.

2. Ese libro ha sido escrito _____ un escritor famoso.

3. La casa fue pintada _____ mi hermano.

    4. Tiene una tarea _____ la mañana.

    5. Trajo el regalo _____ los enfermos.

B. Make augmentatives and diminutives out of the following words.

    1. cara . . . .   6. doctor . . . .

    2. mano . . . .   7. rápido . . . .

    3. bueno . . . .   8. hospital . . . .

    4. malo . . . .   9. profesor . . . .

    5. enfermo . . . .   10. trabajo . . . .

C. Give the proper form of the verbs in the conditional mood.

    1. Me (gustar) _____ dar un paseo.

    2. El doctor (trabajar) _____ con gusto.

    3. Yo (almorzar) _____ allí.

    4. tú (explicar) _____ la lección.

    5. Pepe y yo (ir) _____ más tarde.

D. Write a short composition about the importance of planned parenthood.

E. Have a dialogue with one of your classmates using some of the information given in this lesson.

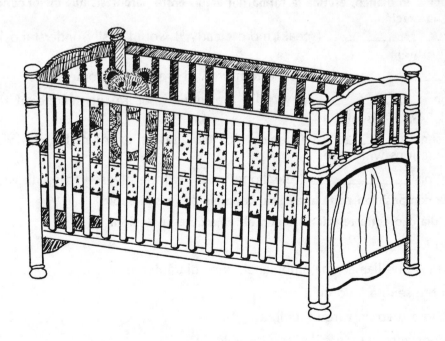

F. Answer in Spanish.

1. ¿Por qué mueren muchos niños en algunos países subdesarrollados? . . . .

. . . .

2. ¿Ha presenciado usted un parto? ¿Cómo le pareció? . . . .

. . . .

3. ¿Cómo es la sala de maternidad en el hospital donde usted trabaja? . . . .

. . . .

4. ¿Qué trabajo hace un médico partero? . . . .

. . . .

5. ¿Por qué ya no hay muchas parteras? . . . .

EJERCICIOS — EXERCISES

(Estudiantes de inglés — Students learning English)

A. Escriba seis oraciones con expresiones de tiempo.

1. . . . .   4. . . . .

2. . . . .   5. . . . .

3. . . . .   6. . . . .

B. Escriba seis oraciones condicionales en el futuro de posibilidad.

1. . . . .   4. . . . .

2. . . . .   5. . . . .

3. . . . .   6. . . . .

C. En los espacios en blanco, escriba la forma del verbo entre paréntesis que mejor concuerde con el resto de la oración.

1. If you _____ (speak) more clearly, I would easily understand how to get to the hospital.

2. If I _____ (have) time tomorrow, I would buy some shoes.

3. If Tom _____ (pay) Julie the money before the second of the month, he won't have to pay interest.

4. If Susan _____ (prepare) for her classes every night, she would pass her examinations with ease.

5. If Joseph _____ (telephone) me, I will be pleased to speak with him.

D. Escriba una composición corta acerca de la paternidad responsable.

E. Escriba un diálogo corto relacionado con el tema de esta lección.

F. Traduzca al inglés.

1. Tenemos que llamar una ambulancia inmediatamente. . . . .

2. La pobre señora tuvo un aborto. . . . .

3. La señora tuvo un varón (hembra). . . . .

4. Es importante la paternidad responsable. . . . .

5. El bebé nació antes de tiempo. . . . .

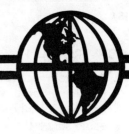

DIET AND NUTRITION
DIETA Y NUTRICION

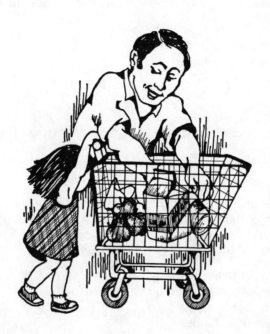

VOCABULARY — VOCABULARIO

A. Medical — Médico

alimentos sin refinar	— unrefined foods	nutrición,	
bajo de azúcar	— low-sugar	alimentación	— nutrition
calorías	— calories	obesidad	— obesity
delgado (a)	— thin	pan integral	— whole grain bread
dieta, régimen	— diet	potasio	— potassium
entre comidas	— in between meals	rico en proteínas	— high-protein
gelatina	— gelatine	sodio	— sodium
grasa, gordo (a)	— fat	suplementos minerales	— mineral suplements

B. General

atractivo	— attractive	modelo	— model
belleza	— beauty	necesitar	— to need
deleitarse, disfrutar	— to enjoy	ordenar, mandar	— to order, command
femenino	— feminine	peso, pesar	— weight, to weigh
mantenerse	— to keep, stay, maintain oneself	rebajar de peso, adelgazar	— to reduce
masculino	— masculine, male	sociedad	— society
mayor	— greater	tener exceso de peso, ser gordo u obeso	— to be overweight, obese, fat
menor	— less, lesser		

CONVERSATION — CONVERSACION

A. A certain school district is facing serious problems, and one of the supervisors, Dr. Carl Marks, who just came from England, has some suggestions to make.

Cierto distrito escolar afronta serios problemas, y uno de los supervisores, el doctor Carl Marks, que acaba de venir de Inglaterra, tiene algunas sugerencias que hacer.

Marks — After examining the problem, I have a suggestion to make.

Después de examinar el problema, tengo una sugerencia que hacer.

Principal — El doctor Marks dice que después de haber examinado el problema tiene una sugerencia que hacer.

A member of the board — ¿Cuál es?

What is it?

Principal — What is it?

Marks — We need a new school diet program.

Necesitamos un programa nuevo de dieta escolar.

Principal — Necesitamos un programa nuevo de dieta escolar.

Marks — From next week on, we'll give the students a high-protein, low-sugar lunch of natural unrefined foods.

Desde la semana entrante en adelante les daremos a los estudiantes un almuerzo rico en proteínas, bajo de azúcar, de alimentos naturales sin refinar.

Principal — Desde la semana entrante en adelante daremos a los estudiantes un almuerzo rico en proteínas, bajo en azúcar, de alimentos naturales y sin refinar.

Another member of the board — ¿Qué hacemos con la comida que ya tenemos?

Principal — What do we do with the food we already have?

Marks — What kind of food?

¿Qué clase de comida?

Principal — ¿Qué clase de comida?

Member — Helados, gaseosas, pasteles, etc.

Ice cream, candy, soft drinks, pies, etc.

Principal — Ice cream, candy, soft drinks, cakes, etc.

Marks — We can get rid of it. We need milk, proteins (meat, poultry, cheese, fish, or eggs) beans, fresh vegetables, fruits, margarine, and whole grain bread.

Podemos deshacernos de ella. Necesitamos leche, proteínas (carne, pollo, queso, pescado o huevos), frijoles, verduras, frutas, margarina y pan integral.

Principal — Podemos deshacernos de ella. Necesitamos leche, proteínas (carne, pollo, queso, pescado o huevos), frijoles, verduras, frutas, margarina y pan integral.

Member of the board — Eso me parece una idea excelente.	*That's seems an excellent idea.*
Other members — Es una buena idea.	*It's a good idea.*
Principal — They agree.	*Están de acuerdo.*
Marks — Let's see how it works.	*Vamos a ver cómo funciona.*
Principal — Vamos a ver cómo funciona.	
Member — Va a funcionar.	
Members — Va a funcionar.	*It's going to work.*

GRAMMATICAL HINTS — APUNTES GRAMATICALES

A. Past participles in Spanish

1. Past participles in Spanish are made by adding the endings **ado** to the stems of verbs ending in **ar**, and **ido** to the stems of verbs ending in **er** and **ir**.

e.g. hablar — habl**ado**
comer — com**ido**
vivir — viv**ido**

2. There are some irregular past participles.

e.g.

ver	— **visto**	escribir	— **escrito**
hacer	— **hecho**	morir	— **muerto**
decir	— **dicho**	imprimir	— **impreso** (imprimido)
poner	— **puesto**	volver	— **vuelto**
soltar	— **suelto**	romper	— **roto**
traer	— **traído**	leer	— **leído**

3. El participio pasado en inglés.

Para tener una información completa véase la lista de participios pasados de verbos irregulares que aparecen en la pág. 93-94. El participio pasado de verbos regulares se forma tal como el pretérito: talk — talk**ed.**

B. Passive voice in Spanish

The Spanish passive voice is used less frequently than the English passive. It is formed by the verb **ser** followed by the past participle, which agrees in gender and number with the subject.

e.g. La América **fue descubierta** por Colón. (**por Colón** indicates the agent.)
La fruta **es comida** por el pájaro.
Los temas **serán desarrollados** por el radiólogo.

C. Active voice in Spanish

If there is an agent in the sentence, it becomes the subject when the passive is changed to the active voice.

e.g. Colón descubrió la América.
El pájaro come la fruta.
El radiólogo desarrollará los temas.

When there is no agent, the reflexive **se** is used.

e.g. El español es hablado — **se** habla español.
El árbol fue cortado — **se** cortó el árbol.

D. La voz activa en inglés

La voz activa se usa cuando el sujeto realiza la acción.
e.g. The patient brings her card — la paciente trae su tarjeta.

E. La voz pasiva en inglés

1. La voz pasiva se usa cuando el sujeto de la oración recibe la acción.
   e.g. The patient is brought by the orderly.

2. La voz pasiva se forma con el auxiliar **to be** y el participio pasado del verbo principal.

Active Voice	Passive Voice
He brings the flowers.	The flowers are brought (by him-el agente).
He brought the flowers.	The flowers were brought by him.
He will bring the flowers.	The flowers will be brought by him.
He has brought the flowers.	The flowers have been brought by him.

F. Whichever, whatever, wherever, whoever, etc.

La terminación **ever** se añade a **what, who, when, which,** para formar palabras compuestas que equivalen a las compuestas con **quiera** en castellano, o a expresiones verbales equivalentes.
e.g. Wherever he goes, everyone likes him — dondequiera que va, todos lo quieren.
   Whoever gets there first is supposed to win a prize — el que llegue primero ganará
                                                                    un premio.
   Don't pay any attention to whatever he says — diga lo que diga, no le hagas caso.

CONVERSATION — CONVERSACION (Cont.)

B. María Ordoñez visits her doctor because she is 30 pounds overweight. Her husband does the translating.

María Ordóñez visita a su doctor porque tiene 30 libras de exceso de peso. Su esposo hace la traducción.

Doctor — What's your problem, Mrs. Ordoñez?	*¿Cuál es su problema, señora Ordóñez?*
Sr. Ordóñez — She is worried about her excess weight.	*Está preocupada por su exceso de peso.*
Doctor — How many meals does she eat a day?	*¿Cuántas comidas come al día?*
Sr. Ordóñez — Three.	*Tres.*
Doctor — Does she eat in between meals?	*¿Come entre comidas?*
Sr. Ordóñez — Once in a while.	*De vez en cuando.*
Doctor — I'm going to put her on a very strict diet so that she will lose those extra pounds, but she has to exercise her will-power.	*Voy a ponerle una dieta rigurosa para que rebaje esas libras de más, pero tiene que ejercitar su fuerza de voluntad.*
Sr. Ordóñez — El doctor te va a poner una dieta rigurosa para que rebajes esas libras de más, pero tienes que ejercitar tu fuerza de voluntad.	
María — ¿Cuál es la dieta?	*What diet is it?*

Sr. Ordóñez — What diet is it?

Doctor — It's diet with little sugar, no grease, no refined foods, and with many vegetables.

Es una dieta con poco azúcar, sin grasa, sin alimentos refinados y con bastantes verduras.

Sr. Ordóñez — Es una dieta con poco azúcar, sin grasa, sin alimentos refinados y con bastantes verduras.

María — ¿Por cuánto tiempo estaré en dieta?

How long will I be on the diet?

Sr. Ordóñez — How long will she be on the diet?

Doctor — We'll see how many pounds she'll lose in the first month.

Veremos cuántas libras perderá en el primer mes.

Sr. Ordóñez — Veremos cuántas libras perderás en el primer mes.

María — Está bien.

COMMENTARY — COMENTARIO

Peter Paul Rubens, the famous Dutch painter, delighted in painting fat people. For him, feminine beauty consisted of fat. A beautiful woman had to be at least 50 pounds overweight. His models, of course, would not be acceptable in our times. Nowadays to keep oneself slim is the great preoccupation of our society and almost everyone wants to lose weight.

Pedro Pablo Rubens, el famoso pintor holandés, se deleitaba pintando personas gordas. Para él, la belleza femenina consistía en la gordura. Una mujer hermosa tenía que tener por lo menos unas 50 libras de exceso de peso. Sus modelos, desde luego, no serían muy aceptados en nuestros días. En la actualidad mantenerse delgado es la gran preocupación de nuestra sociedad y casi todo el mundo quiere perder peso.

Questions:

1. Who was Rubens?
2. What did he like to paint?
3. According to Rubens, what did feminine beauty consist of?
4. What does our society think of fat today?
5. What do many people want to do?

Preguntas:

1. ¿Quién fue Rubens?
2. ¿Qué le gustaba pintar?
3. ¿En qué consistía, según él, la belleza femenina?
4. ¿Qué piensa hoy día nuestra sociedad de la gordura?
5. ¿Qué quieren hacer muchas personas?

ADDITIONAL INFORMATION — INFORMACION ADICIONAL

1. Weights and measures — Pesos y medidas

acre	— acre	metro cúbico	— cubic meter
centímetro	— centimeter, centimetre	milímetro	— millimeter, millimetre
decímetro	— decimeter, decimetre	milla	— mile
estadio	— furlong	milla cuadrada	— square mile
galón	— gallon	milla náutica	— knot
gramo	— gram, gramme	onza	— ounce (oz.)
hectárea	— hectare	pie	— foot
hectogramo	— hectogram	pie cúbico	— cubic foot
kilogramo	— kilogram	pulgada	— inch
kilómetro	— kilometer	pulgada cúbica	— cubic inch
libra	— pound (lb.)	tonelada	— ton
litro	— liter, litre	tonelada métrica	— metric ton
metro	— meter, metre	un cuarto de galón	— quart
		yarda	— yard

2. Spanish last names   Apellidos ingleses

Alvarez	Ocampo	Carpenter	Cole
Alva	Ortega	Carter	Collins
Arano	Peinado	Case	Cook
Cardozo	Romero	Chapman	Crane
Garnica	Rosas	Clark	Davis
Gutiérrez	Vargas	Cochran	Day
Jiménez	Venegas		
Marino	Ulloa		

3. Useful expressions — Expresiones útiles

Abundancia de la vitamina B	— abundance of vitamin B
Buena salud	— good health
Coma una comida completa	— Eat a full meal.
Debe aumentar de peso	— You should gain weight.
Debe controlar el peso	— You should control your weight.
Debe perder algunas libras	— You should lose some pounds.
Debe seguir una dieta especial	— You should follow a special diet.
Está demasiado pesado	— You are overweight.
Hay gente desnutrida	— There are undernourished people.
Píldoras para reducir	— reducing pills
Pobre en vitaminas	— poor in vitamines
Problemas de la personalidad	— personality problems
Pruebe otras clases diferentes	— Try different kinds
Rica en proteínas	— rich in proteins
Una dieta balanceada	— a balanced diet
Una variedad de comida	— a variety of food

4. Idiomatic expressions — Expresiones idiomáticas

Al romper el día	— at daybreak	Digno de confianza	— trustworthy
Cuesta abajo	— downhill	Echarlo todo a rodar	— to upset everything carelessly
Cuesta arriba	— uphill		
De trecho en trecho	— at intervals	En buena hora	— luckily

| Estoy muy aburrido | — I am bored to death | Mirar de hito en hito | — to stare at |
| Hacer cola | — to line up, stand in line | Sin medida | — to excess |

5. Expressions with the reflexive "se" — Expresiones con "se"

Se alquila un tocadiscos	— Record Player for Rent	Se necesita una secretaria bilingüe	— Bilingual Secretary Needed
Se alquilan embarcaciones	— Boats for Rent	Se ponen inyecciones	— Injections Given Here
Se dan clases de francés	— French Taught Here	Se prohibe comer en este lugar	— No Food Permitted
Se compra oro y plata	— We Buy Gold and Silver	Se prohibe fijar carteles	— Post no Bills
		Se prohibe fumar	— No Smoking
Se habla español	— Spanish Spoken	Se prohibe pescar	— No Fishing
Se hacen traducciones aquí	— Translations Done Here	Se venden periódicos	— Newspaper for Sale

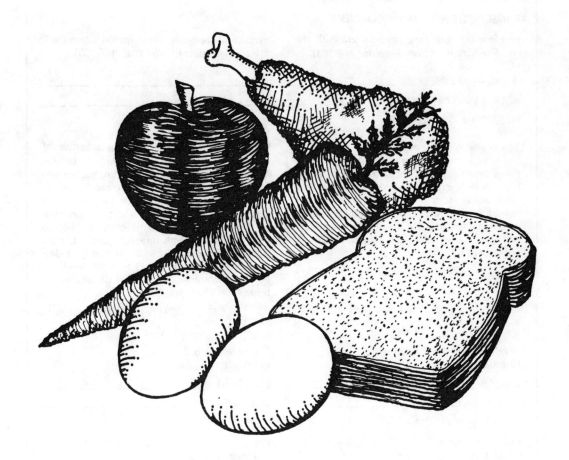

6. The Lung-El pulmón

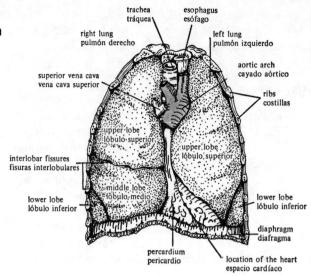

trachea
tráquea

esophagus
esófago

right lung
pulmón derecho

left lung
pulmón izquierdo

superior vena cava
vena cava superior

aortic arch
cayado aórtico

ribs
costillas

upper lobe
lóbulo superior

upper lobe
lóbulo superior

interlobar fissures
fisuras interlobulares

lower lobe
lóbulo inferior

middle lobe
lóbulo medio

lower lobe
lóbulo inferior

diaphragm
diafragma

percardium
pericardio

location of the heart
espacio cardíaco

BILINGUAL PROJECT — PROYECTO BILINGUE

TRANSCRIPTION — TRANSCRIPCION

Complete the following report along with the completed transcription. (See pp. 107-108).

Prepare la siguiente transcripción y termine los informes adjuntos. (Vea pág. 107-108).

NAME — NOMBRE: _____

ADDRESS — DIRECCION:_____

SITUATION — SITUACION:

This 6 year-old boy was admitted to the Ear, Nose, and Throat Department of the hospital for surgery because of repeated ear infections. His ears were drained and infected tissue was removed in surgery. The pathology report indicated chronic infection without evidence of any malignancy. He did well after surgery and was subsequently discharged to further out-patient follow-up.

Este niño de 6 años de edad fue admitido al Departamento de Otorrinolaringología del hospital para ser sometido a un tratamiento quirúrgico a causa de tener repetidas infecciones en el oído. Se le practicó un drenaje de los oídos y se le extripó durante la operación un tejido infectado. El informe patológico indicó que tenía una infección crónica, pero sin evidencia de malignidad. Le fue bien después de la operación y más adelante fue dado de alta, pero tenía que regresar periódicamente para un chequeo.

SEQUENCE OF REPORTS   —   ORDEN DE LOS INFORMES:

A—1

History and Physical Exam
Historia y examen físico

Completed _____

Terminado _____

A—2

Operative Record
Informe quirúrgico

Completed _____

Terminado _____

A—3

Pathology Report
Informe patológico

Completed _____

Terminado _____

A—4

Clinical Resumé
Resumen clínico

Completed _____

Terminado _____

EXERCISES — EJERCICIOS

(Students learning Spanish — Estudiantes de español)

A. Give the past participle of each of the following verbs.

1. comer ....
2. devolver ....
3. deponer ....
4. comprar ....
5. ser ....

6. tener ....
7. contradecir ....
8. ir ....
9. reimprimir ....
10. deshacer ....

B. Change the following sentences from active to passive voice.

1. La enfermera trae la medicina. ....
2. Los pacientes comen la comida. ....
3. Los técnicos sacan las radiografías. ....
4. El farmacéutico prepara la receta. ....
5. Los enfermeros pagan la cuenta. ....

C. Change the following sentences from passive to active voice.

1. Los medicamentos fueron entregados por el trabajador. ....
2. La operación es hecha por el cirujano. ....
3. El libro es traducido por el profesor. ....
4. Las vitaminas son vendidas. ....
5. La dieta será seguida por el paciente. ....

D. Write a short composition using the passive voice.

E. Plan a diabetic diet. (See Chapter 3, additional information about food).

F. Answer in complete Spanish sentences.

1. ¿Cuántas libras pesa Ud? ....
2. ¿Cuántas libras le gustaría pesar? ....
3. ¿Qué dieta le recomendaría Ud. a una persona que tiene un problema con la gordura? ....
   ....
4. ¿Por qué es importante una dieta sin grasa? ....
5. ¿Cómo afecta la gordura al corazón? ....

EJERCICIOS — EXERCISES

(Estudiantes de inglés — Students learning English)

A. Cámbiense las siguientes oraciones a la voz pasiva.

1. The doctor performed the operation. ....
2. The nurse brings the medicine. ....
3. The patients eat the food. ....
4. The technician takes the X-rays. ....
5. The pharmacist prepares the prescription. ....

B. Cámbiense las siguientes oraciones a la voz activa.

1. The book was written by Shakespeare. ....
2. The medicine was brought by the orderly. ....
3. The operation was performed by the surgeon. ....
4. The vitamins are sold by the pharmacist. ....
5. The newspaper is delivered by the delivery boy. ....

C. Escriba seis oraciones con whichever, whatever, wherever y whoever.

1. ....   4. ....
2. ....   5. ....
3. ....   6. ....

D. Prepare una dieta para un diabético. (Para mayor información vea la pág. 24).

E. Traduzca las siguientes oraciones al inglés.

1. Yo quiero rebajar 20 libras. ....
2. El tiene exceso de peso. ....
3. Buscan una dieta balanceada. ....
4. Hay que suprimir las grasas y los dulces. ....
5. Las golosinas entre comidas son malas. ....

F. Conteste las siguientes preguntas en inglés.

1. How many meals do you eat a day? ....
2. How much do you weigh? ....
3. What's your height? ....
4. Are you a vegetarian? ....
5. Who is the dietician in your hospital? ....

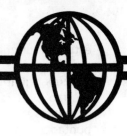

SURGERY
CIRUGIA

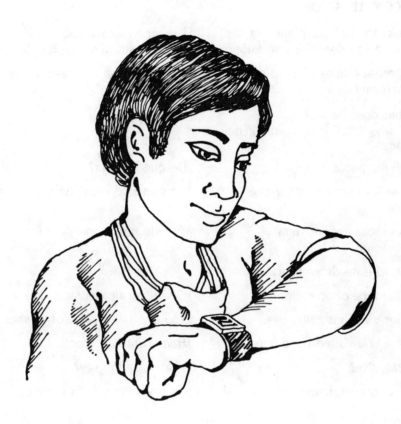

VOCABULARY — VOCABULARIO

A. Medical — Médico

anestesia local	— local anesthetic	histerectomía	— hysterectomy
anestesiólogo	— anesthesiologist	laparatomía	— laparatomy
apéndice	— appendix	mastectomía	— mastectomy
biopsia	— biopsy	operación quirúrgica,	
cirugía	— surgery	cirugía	— surgical operation
cirujano	— surgeon	ovarios	— ovaries
componer una fractura	— to set a fracture	riñón	— kidney
desinfectar	— to disinfect	tumor	— tumor
dilatar la uretra	— to dilate the urethra	útero	— uterus
fibroma	— fibroma	vasectomía	— vasectomy

B. General

afeitar	— to shave	cráneo	— cranium
amputar	— to amputate	defectuoso (a)	— defective

extirpar, suprmir	— to extirpate, remove	quiste	— cyst
guardar	— to keep	quitar, suprimir	— to remove
película orientadora	— orientation film	quitarse	— to take off
postizo	— false	ramo, rama	— branch, division
preguntas	— questions	reparar los tejidos	— to repair tissues
puntadas	— stitches		

CONVERSATION—CONVERSACION

A. Mr. Montoya talks to the receptionist in the hospital; his son George does the translating.

El señor Montoya habla con la recepcionista del hospital, su hijo George le ayuda a traducir.

Montoya — Señorita, éste es un caso de emergencia.

Miss, this is an emergency case.

Receptionist — What does he say?

¿Qué dice?

George — He says that this is an emergency case.

Receptionist — Tell me about it.

¿De qué se trata?

George — La señorita quiere saber qué pasa.

She wants to know what is wrong.

Montoya — Mi esposa necesita una operación.

My wife needs an operation.

George — His wife needs an operation.

Receptionist — What type of operation?

¿Qué clase de operación?

George — I think she has gallstones.

Creo que tiene cálculos biliares.

Receptionist — Have you visited the doctor?

¿Han visitado al doctor?

Montoya — ¿Qué dice?

What does she say?

George — Dice que si hemos visitado al doctor.

She is wondering if we have visited the doctor.

Montoya — Dile que lo hemos visto varias veces, y que él dice que necesita una operación.

Tell her we've seen him several times and he says she needs an operation.

George — We have seen him several times and he says she needs an operation.

Receptionist — Who is your doctor?

¿Quién es su doctor?

George — Dr. Herman.

Receptionist — Bring her over then.

Tráigala entonces.

George — We'll bring her tomorrow because her surgery will be the day after tomorrow.

La traeremos mañana porque la cirugía será pasado mañana.

Receptionist — All right. We'll have everything ready for her.

Muy bien. Tendremos todo listo para ella.

GRAMMATICAL HINTS—APUNTES GRAMATICALES

A. Present perfect tense in Spanish

The present perfect tense is formed from the present of **haber** plus the past participle.

e.g. hemos hablado, comido, visto, etc.
has   hablado, comido, visto, etc.
ha   hablado, comido, visto, etc.
hemos hablado, comido, visto, etc.
han   hablado, comido, visto, etc.
He viajado dos veces por Europa — I have traveled twice in Europe.

B. Pluperfect or past perfect

The pluperfect tense is formed from the imperfect of **haber** plus the past participle.

e.g. había   hecho
habías   hecho
había   hecho
habíamos hecho
habían   hecho
Cuando ví a Juan, ya había vendido su auto — When I saw John, he had already sold the car.

C. El presente perfecto en inglés

1. El presente perfecto se forma con las formas del verbo **to have** en el presente de indicativo y el participio pasado.
e.g. I have talked too much — he hablado demasiado.
I have paid for it   — lo he pagado.

2. Se pueden usar contracciones, afirmativas y negativas, en las oraciones del presente perfecto.
e.g. I've talked too much   — he hablado demasiado.
I've paid for it   — lo he pagado.
We haven't decided   — no hemos decidido.

3. La lista de participios pasados irregulares se halla en la lección 10, pág. 93-94.

4. En preguntas el participio va al final.
e.g. Where have the doctors been? — ¿dónde han estado los doctores?

5. El pluscuamperfecto

El pluscuamperfecto se forma con el verbo **to have** en el pretérito y el participio pasado.
e.g. I had talked   — había hablado.
Mary told me that she had bought the car — Mary me dijo que había comprado el carro.

CONVERSATION — CONVERSACION (Cont.)

B. Jack Ross será operado en la mañana y recibe una orientación breve la noche anterior. Mary Jones hace la traducción.

Jack Ross will have surgery in the morning, and he receives a brief orientation the night before. Mary Jones does the translating.

Enfermera — Señor Ross, como mañana será su operación queremos que vea una película orientadora esta noche.

Mr. Ross, since your operation is tomorrow, we would like you to watch an orientation film tonight.

Mary   — Mr. Ross, since your operation is tomorrow, we would like for you

	to watch an orientation film tonight.	
Jack	— Whatever you say.	*Como digan.*
Enfermera	— Antes de la película nos gustaría hacerle algunas preguntas.	*Before the film we'd like to ask you some questions.*
Mary	— Before the film we'd like to ask you some questions.	
Jack	— At your service.	*A sus órdenes.*
Enfermera	— Pregúnteselas en inglés	*Ask them in English.*
Mary	— Have you ever had surgery before?	*¿Ha tenido una operación antes?*
Jack	— No, this is my first.	*No, ésta es la primera.*
Mary	— Do you have anything artificial (false) we can keep for you?	*¿Tiene algo postizo que podemos guardarle?*
Jack	— Yes, my dentures, my hairpiece, and I would like you to keep my rings and my watch.	*Sí, mis dientes postizos, la peluca, y quisiera que me guardara mis anillos y el reloj.*
Mary	— ¿Qué más le digo?	*What else should I tell him?*
Enfermera	— Dile que tiene que firmar el permiso para la operación.	*Tell him he has to sign the release form for the surgery.*
Mary	— Now you have to sign the release form for the surgery.	
Jack	— All right.	
Mary	— That's all, now let's watch the orientation film.	*Eso es todo, ahora vamos a ver la película orientadora.*

GRAMMATICAL HINTS — APUNTES GRAMATICALES

D. Negatives in Spanish

1. In a negative sentence **no** or some other negative word precedes the verb.
e.g. No veo a nadie — I don't see anybody.

2. Double negatives are allowed in Spanish.
e.g. **No** tengo **nada.**

3. Affirmative and **Negative** words

alguien	— something	nada	— nothing
alguien	— someone	nadie	— nobody, no one
alguno	— someone	ninguno	— nobody, no one
siempre	— always	nunca, jamás	— never
también	— also	tampoco	— not (nor) ... either
y	— and	ni	— neither... nor, not... or, not.

e.g. La casa no es **ni** nueva **ni** grande — The house in **neither** new **nor** large.

4. Jamás may also mean **ever.**
e.g. ¿Ha estado Ud. jamás en México? — Have you ever been in Mexico?

E. Negativos en inglés

En inglés no se usa el doble negativo como en español.
e.g. We don't have anything — No tenemos nada.

COMMENTARY — COMENTARIO

Surgery is a very important branch of medicine and every day it is becoming more popular. Surgery is practiced when an extremity of the body needs to be amputated or in order to remove a defective organ; it is also useful for the removal of an appendix that has become inflamed or to eliminate some part of the body that has been infected by cancer. Today this science is being perfected more and more since surgery is being done on the heart, on the brain, on the eyes, and on many other parts of the body. That is why surgery plays such a very important role in modern medicine.

La cirugía es una rama muy importante de la medicina y cada día tiene mayor acogida. Se practica la cirugía cuando hay que amputar un miembro del cuerpo o eliminar órganos defectuosos; también sirve para extirpar una apéndice que está inflamada o para eliminar alguna parte del cuerpo infectada por el cáncer. Hoy en día esta ciencia se está perfeccionando cada vez más pues se practican operaciones en el corazón, en el cerebro, en los ojos y en muchas otras partes del cuerpo. Es por eso que la cirugía es de tan gran importancia en la medicina moderna.

Questions:

1. Why is surgery important?
2. What types of surgery are done?
3. When is surgery applied?
4. Why is it a very delicate profession?
5. What is done with an inflamed appendix?

Preguntas:

1. ¿Por qué es importante la cirugía?
2. ¿Qué clase de operaciones se practican?
3. ¿Cuándo se practica la cirugía?
4. ¿Por qué es una profesión muy delicada?
5. ¿Qué se hace con una apéndice inflamada?

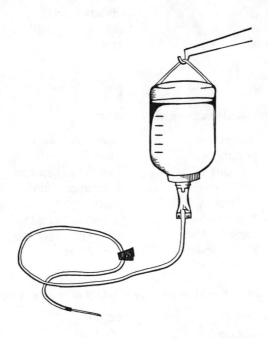

ADDITIONAL INFORMATION — INFORMACION ADICIONAL

1. Nationalities — Nacionalidades

alemán	— German	hindú	— Indian (Hindu)
americano	— American	holandés	— Dutch
árabe	— Arabian	irlandés	— Irish
argentino	— Argentinian	italiano	— Italian
austríaco	— Austrian	japonés	— Japanese
belga	— Belgian	mexicano	— Mexican
brasileño	— Brazilian	noruego	— Norwegian
británico	— British	persa, iraní	— Persian, Iranian
búlgaro	— Bulgarian	polaco	— Polish
canadiense	— Canadian	portugués	— Portuguese
colombiano	— Colombian	rumano	— Rumanian
cubano	— Cuban	ruso	— Russian
checo	— Czechoslovakian, Czechoslovak	sudafricano	— South African
		sudamericano	— South American
chino	— Chinese	sueco	— Swedish
danés	— Danish	suizo	— Swiss
egipcio	— Egyptian	turco	— Turkish
escosés	— Scotch, Scottish	yugoslavo	— Yugoslav, Yugoslavian
finlandés	— Finnish		
francés	— French		
griego	— Greek		

2. Spanish last names / Apellidos ingleses

Anaya	Franco	Douglas	Edwards
Barbosa	Gil	Downs	Elliot
Barros	Hurtado	Duncan	Ellyson
Benítez	León	Dunford	Emmerson
Bustos	Mendoza	Dunlap	Evans
Carrillo	Montiel	Estman	Evanson
Carvajal	Salazar		
Casas	Santos		
Corona	Urbina		

3. Some medicines and drugs — Medicamentos y drogas

analgésicos	— analgesics	laxantes, purgantes	— laxatives
anestésicos	— anesthetics	narcóticos	— narcotics
antiácidos	— antacids	píldoras, pastillas, comprimidos	— pills, tablets
antibióticos	— antibiotics		
antisépticos	— antiseptics	sedantes, tranquilizantes, calmantes	— sedatives, tranquilizers
astringentes	— astringents		
cápsulas	— capsules		
descongestionantes	— descongestants	ungüentos	— unguents, salves, ointments
estimulantes	— stimulants		

4. Parts of the body commonly requiring surgery — Organos que a menudo necesitan cirugía

amígdalas	— tonsils	colon	— colon
cáncer	— cancer	corazón	— heart
cataratas	— cataracts	garganta	— throat
cerebro	— brain	hemorroides	— hemorrhoids

hernia	— hernia	tiroides	— thyroid
intestino	— intestine	úlcera	— ulcer
páncreas	— pancreas	vesícula biliar	— gallbladder
próstata	— prostate		

5. Useful expressions — Expresiones útiles

Las cirugías mayores me fascinan	— Major surgery fascinates me.
Le vamos a operar las amígdalas	— We're going to operate on your tonsils.
Ser buen cirujano requiere gran habilidad	— Great ability is required to become a good surgeon.
Se han practicado muchas cirugías innecesarias	— Many unnecessary operations have been performed.
¿Qué operación me va a hacer?	— What operation are you going to do on me?
El anestesiólogo siempre está ocupado	— The anesthesiologist is always busy.
Le vamos a hacer una operación exploratoria	— We're going to do an exploratory operation.
Nadie puede entrar a la sala de operaciones sin autorización previa	— No one can enter the operation room without previous authorization.
La doctora Gómez es una buena cirujana	— Dr. Gómez is a good surgeon.
Le vamos a quitar los puntos	— We're going to remove the stitches.

6. Idiomatic expressions — Expresiones idiomáticas

a las mil maravillas	— wonderfully well
Amanecerá y veremos	— Time will tell.
de ahora en adelante	— from now on
El doctor quiere verlo la semana próxima	— The doctor wants to see you next week.
Eso sólo faltaba	— That's all I needed.
la verdad clara y desnuda	— the truth pure and simple
la mayor parte (la mayoría) de	— the majority (the greater part)
por lo general	— on an (the) average
sea como fuere (sea)	— be that as it may
¿Sufre de cardialgia (pirosis)?	— Do you have heartburn (cardialgia)?
tarde o temprano	— sooner or later

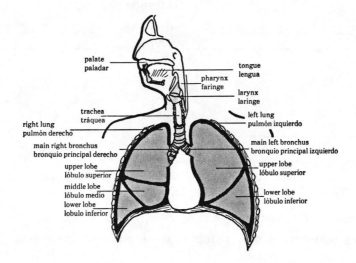

BILINGUAL PROJECT — PROYECTO BILINGUE

TRANSCRIPTION — TRANSCRIPCION

Complete the following report along with the completed transcription. (See pp. 107-108).

Prepare la siguiente transcripción y termine los informes adjuntos. (Vea pág. 107-108).

NAME — NOMBRE: _____

ADDRESS — DIRECCION: _____

SITUATION — SITUACION:

This 63 year-old patient was admitted to the hospital with urinary retention. His medical history was reviewed and an initial evaluation done. X-ray studies helped in arriving at diagnosis and surgery was deemed necessary to relieve his urinary obstruction. The tissue removed was benign. His hospital stay and convalescence were uneventful and he was discharged after a short time.

Un paciente de 63 años de edad fue admitido al hospital por sufrir de retención de la orina. Se repasó su historia médica y se le hizo una evaluación inicial. Un estudio radiográfico ayudó a dictar un diagnóstico y se decidió que se necesitaba una operación para extirparle el tejido que obstruía. El tejido que se le extirpó resultó ser benigno. Su estadía en el hospital y su convalescencia resultaron sin contratiempo alguno y al poco tiempo fue dado de alta.

SEQUENCE OF REPORTS   —   ORDEN DE LOS INFORMES:

A—1

History and Physical Exam
Historia y examen físico

Completed _____

Terminado _____

A—2

X-ray Report
Informe radiológico

Completed _____

Terminado _____

A—3

Operative Record
Informe quirúrgico

Completed _____
Terminado _____

A—4

Pathology Report
Informe patológico

Completed _____
Terminado _____

A—5

Clinical Resumé
Resumen clínico

Completed _____

Terminado _____

EXERCISES — EJERCICIOS

(Students learning Spanish — Estudiantes de español)

A. Change the following sentences into sentences in the present perfect tense.

1. El radiólogo saca la placa. ....

2. Los pacientes comen el desayuno. ....

3. El cirujano realiza la operación. ....

4. El farmacéutico prepara la receta. ....

5. Ernestina trabaja en la sala de emergencia. ....

B. Change the same sentences of exercise A into sentences in the pluperfect.

1. ....

2. ....

3. ....

4. ....

5. ....

C. Change the following sentences into negative sentences.

1. El enfermero salió también. ....

2. El hospital es bueno y barato. ....

3. Los pacientes son muy disciplinados. ....

4. ¿Hay algún restaurante en este lugar? ....

5. ¿Tienes algo bueno? ....

D. Write a composition in Spanish about the importance of surgery.

....
....
....
....
....
....
....
....
....
....

E. Answer in Spanish.

1. ¿Qué clase de operación ha visto usted? ....

2. ¿Qué opina usted de los transplantes de corazón? ....

3. ¿Cómo se puede detener una hemorragia? ....

4. ¿Qué papel desempeña la anestesia? ....

5. ¿Qué países le gustaría conocer? ....

EJERCICIOS — EXERCISES

(Estudiantes de inglés — Students learning English)

A. Vuelva a escribir las siguientes oraciones, cambiando el tiempo del verbo al presente perfecto.

1. The doctor works at the hospital. ....
2. The patients sleep well. ....
3. The nurse walks to work. ....
4. The technician prepares prescriptions. ....
5. The drugstore is opened on Sundays. ....

B. Transforme las oraciones del ejercicio A a oraciones en el pluscuamperfecto.

1. ....
2. ....
3. ....
4. ....
5. ....

C. Traduzca al inglés.

1. La enfermera ha trabajado toda la noche. ....
2. ¿Qué dijo el doctor? ....
3. El paciente había tomado la sopa. ....
4. La farmacia vende medicinas. ....
5. La planificación familiar es importante. ....

D. Cambie las siguientes oraciones a la forma negativa.

1. I like school. ....
2. We have some friends. ....
3. He studied hard last night. ....
4. He is going to have a surgery tomorrow. ....
5. Somebody came. ....

E. Conteste en inglés.

1. When was the last time you saw the doctor? ....
2. What kind of operation did you have? ....
3. What kind of work do you do? ....
4. When are you going to watch an operation? ....
5. Who is the man who came with your sister? ....

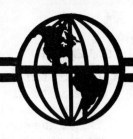

THE NEURO-PSYCHIATRIC UNIT
LA UNIDAD NEUROSIQUIATRICA

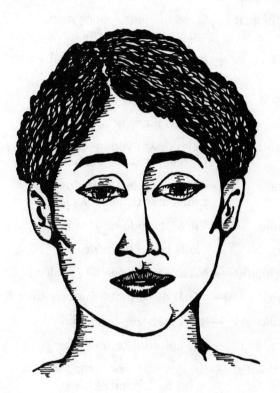

VOCABULARY — VOCABULARIO

A. Medical — Médico

ansiedad	— anxiety
camisa de fuerza	— strait jacket
demencia senil	— senile dementia
desvelo	— wakefulness
dosis excesiva	— overdose
esquizofrenia	— schizophrenia
histerismo	— hysteria
insomnio	— insomnia
loco, demente	— insane, crazy, demented
locura	— insanity
manicomio, asilo de locos	— insane asylum, hospital for the insane
parálisis infantil	— infantile paralysis, poliomyelitis
siquiatra	— psychiatrist
siquiatría	— psychiatry
soporífero	— soporific, sleep-producing drug
suicidio	— suicide
terapia intensiva	— intensive therapy

B. General

aburrido (a)	— bored	efectivo	— real, effective
definición	— definition	entonces	— then
depender	— to depend	hereditario	— hereditary
depresivo, deprimente	— depressive, depressing	incapacitado	— incapacitated
		libro de texto	— textbook
diversos	— several	montón	— pile
editorial	— editorial	por ciento	— per cent

CONVERSATION — CONVERSACION

A. Camilo Torres was taken to the hospital because he had tried to commit suicide by taking an overdose of sleeping pills. Flora Dunca, the nurse, saved his life, and then the psychiatrist talked to him. Flora translated.

Camilo Torres fue llevado al hospital porque había intentado quitarse la vida al tomar una dosis excesiva de píldoras soporíferas. Flora Duncan, la enfermera, le salvó la vida y ahora el siquiatra habla con él. Flora traduce.

Psychiatrist	— Good morning, young man, what's your problem?	*Buenos días, joven, ¿cuál es su problema?*
Flora	— Buenos días, joven, ¿cuál es su problema?	
Camilo	— Tengo muchos problemas.	*I have many problems.*
Flora	— He has many problems.	
Psychiatrist	— Calm down, young man, all problems have a solution.	*Cálmese, joven, todos los problemas tienen solución.*
Flora	— Cálmese joven, todos los problemas tienen solución.	
Camilo	— Estoy aburrido de la vida.	*I am bored with life.*
Flora	— He is bored with life.	
Psychiatrist	— What's your specific problem?	
Flora	— ¿Cuál es su problema específico?	
Camilo	— Un desengaño amoroso.	*An unfortunate love affair.*
Flora	— An unfortunate love afair.	
Psychiatrist	— Is this the first time you have tried to commit suicide?	*¿Es la primera vez que intenta suicidarse?*
Flora	— ¿Es la primera vez que intenta suicidarse?	
Camilo	— La primera.	*The first.*
Flora	— The first.	
Psychiatrist	— You have been very lucky. They brought you to the hospital just in time.	*Ha tenido suerte. Lo trajeron justo a tiempo al hospital.*
Flora	— Ha tenido suerte. Lo trajeron justo a tiempo al hospital.	
Camilo	— Doctor, ¿cómo podré liberarme de esas tendencias suicidas?	*Doctor, how can I get rid of these suicidal tendencies?*
Flora	— He is wondering how he can get rid of his suicidal tendencies?	
Psychiatrist	— Young man, that's up to you. All kinds of mentally ill patients come to this hospital and we try to help each one of them.	*Joven, todo depende de usted. A este hospital llegan enfermos mentales de todas clases y a todos tratamos de ayudarles.*

Flora	— Eso depende de usted. A este hospital llega toda clase de enfermos y a todos tratamos de ayudarles.	
Camilo	— ¿Me ayudarán a mí?	*Will you help me?*
Flora	— Can we help him?	
Psychiatrist	— Of course. That's why we are here.	*Por supuesto. Para eso estamos aquí.*
Flora	— Por supuesto. Para eso estamos aquí.	
Camilo	— Muchas gracias.	

GRAMMATICAL HINTS — APUNTES GRAMATICALES

A. Present subjunctive in Spanish

1. The present subjunctive of all but six verbs is formed by changing the ending of the first person singular of the present indicative as follows:

hablar	comer	vivir	tener	pensar
(hablo)	(como)	(vivo)	(tengo)	(pienso)
hable	coma	viva	tenga	piense
es	as	as	as	es
e	a	a	a	e
emos	amos	amos	amos	emos
en	an	an	an	en

2. The six exceptions are: dar (doy – dé), estar (estoy – esté), haber (he – haya), ir (voy – vaya), saber (sé – sepa), and ser (soy – sea).

ser	ir	dar	saber	estar
sea	vaya	dé	sepa	esté
seas	vayas	des	sepas	estés
sea	vaya	dé	sepa	esté
seamos	vayamos	denos	sepamos	estemos
sean	vayan	den	sepan	estén

B. El subjuntivo en inglés

El subjuntivo se usa bastante en español y es fácil identificarlo. En inglés, al contrario, aunque sí se usa, hay pocas formas peculiares que lo identifiquen. En seguida se presentan tres casos en que sí se puede identificar:

1. Contrario a los hechos.
e.g. If I **were** you I would do the same thing — Si yo fuera usted haría lo mismo.
If I **had** the money, I would buy the car — Si yo tuviera el dinero, compraría el automóvil.

2. Declaraciones de deseos que no son posibles.
e.g. I **wish** he **were** my doctor — ojalá que el fuera mi doctor.

3. En cláusulas seguidas por verbos de petición, demanda y recomendación.
e.g. I recommend that he **take** the medicine — recomiendo que tome la medicina.
I recommended that he **take** the medicine — recomendé que tomara la medicina.

CONVERSATION — CONVERSACION (Cont.)

B. In the Mental Health class the professor is asking some questions of the students, but two of them prefer to answer in Spanish although they understand the questions in English.

En la clase de Salud Mental el profesor les hace algunas preguntas a los alumnos, pero dos de ellos prefieren contestar en español aunque entienden las preguntas en inglés.

Professor — Elena, could you mention some causes of insanity?

Helena, ¿pudiera mencionar algunas causas de locura?

Elena — Hay muchas, tales como trastornos nerviosos, divorcios, problemas en el hogar, fracasos en los estudios, problemas financieros, desengaños amorosos y algunas más.

There are many, such as mental distress, divorces, problems at home, failing at school, money problems, disappointments in love, and several more.

Professor — It sounds correct to me. Joe, explain the roll that insane asylums perform.

Me parece correcto. Joe, explique el papel que desempeñan los manicomios.

Joe — Professor, an insane asylum or hospital for the insane is a place where they keep and treat insane patients.

Profesor, un manicomio o asilo de locos es un lugar donde guardan y tratan a los pacientes con problemas mentales.

Professor — Good. Rosa, what does schizophrenia consist of?

Bien. Rosa, ¿en qué consiste la esquizofrenia?

Rosa — Yo no sé.

I don't know.

Professor — Don't you know? Then look up the definition of that illness in your textbook.

¿No sabe? Busque entonces la definición de esa enfermedad en su libro de texto.

Rosa — Así lo haré.

Professor — Ernest, why is mental health so important?

Ernest, ¿por qué es la salud mental tan importante?

Ernest — Because it helps people with mental problems.

Porque ayuda a las personas con problemas mentales.

Professor — Good. Now I want everyone to write the answers to the following questions.

Bien. Ahora quiero que todos escriban las respuestas a las siguientes preguntas.

Questions

1. Why is syphilis so dangerous?

2. How come there are so many people with nervous breakdown?

3. What do you think of group therapy?

4. Would you recommend that a person who has mental illness watch televisión? Explain your answer.

5. Do you believe that mental illness is hereditary?

Preguntas

¿Por qué es la sífilis tan peligrosa?

¿Por qué hay tantas personas con trastornos nerviosos?

¿Qué opina usted de la terapia en grupo?

¿Le recomendaría mirar televisión a una persona que sufre de una enfermedad mental? Explique su respuesta.

¿Cree usted que la locura es hereditaria?

6. What's the best medicine for insanity?   *¿Cuál es el mejor remedio para la locura?*

7. Do you know anyone who suffers from this type of illness?   *¿Conoce usted a alguien que sufra de este tipo de mal?*

8. Where is the nearest insane asylum.   *¿Dónde está el manicomio más cercano?*

9. What is a psychiatrist?   *¿Qué es un siquiatra?*

10. What is the difference between an insane person and an idiot?   *¿Cuál es la diferencia entre un loco y un idiota?*

GRAMMATICAL HINTS — APUNTES GRAMATICALES (Cont.)

C. Commands in Spanish (The Imperative)

1. The third person forms of the present subjunctive are used with usted (Ud.) to form the imperative (commands).

   Hable (Ud.)   No hable (Ud.)
   Hablen (Uds.)   No hablen (Uds.)

2. The first person plural of the present subjunctive is used to form the imperative whose translation is **Let's** plus an infinitive.
   e.g. Comamos en ese restaurante — Let's eat in that restaurant.

3. This command in also formed with the present indicative of **ir** (with the preposition **a**) plus a verb in the infinitive.
   Comamos — Vamos a comer   Levantémonos — Vamos a levantarnos.

D. El imperativo en inglés

1. El imperativo se forma usando el verbo y omitiendo el sujeto.
   e.g. Close the door! (La admiración no tiene que ponerse siempre).
   Give me the medicine. (Nótese que el pronombre va después).

2. En la forma negativa se pone el verbo auxiliar primero.
   e.g. Don't close the door.
   Do not close the door (para dar más énfasis al mandato).

3. A veces una prohibición toma una forma distinta.
   e.g. No smoking   — no fumar
   No parking   — no estacionarse
   No fishing   — se prohibe pescar
   No trespassing — no traspasar (la propiedad)

4. Un mandato se suaviza cuando se le pone **please** al principio o al final de la petición.
   e.g. Please open your mouth.
   Don't close the door, please.

   Los imperativos de la primera persona del plural se forman anteponiendo **Let's,** ya sea en la forma positiva o negativa.
   e.g. Let's go — vamos.
   Let's not study together tonight — no estudiemos juntos esta noche.

E. Personas o cosas indefinidas en inglés

anybody   — cualquiera, (sea) quien sea   anyone   — cualquiera, (sea) quien sea

anything	— cualquier cosa, (sea) lo que sea	none	— ninguno, nada, nadie
each one	— cada uno	no one	— nadie, ninguno
everyone	— todo el mundo	somebody	— alguien, alguno
everything	— todo	someone	— alguien, alguno
nobody	— ninguno, nadie		

COMMENTARY — COMENTARIO

A certain newspaper editorial said recently that one out of every ten people in this country has suffered from insanity or some mental disturbance at some time in his or her life. The commentator insisted that 48 per cent of the hospital beds are occupied by people that are mentally disturbed. He also considered that the mentally disturbed are increasing in number with the passage of time and the increase of civilization. That is why, according to the writer of the editorial, there should be more emphasis on intensive therapy and at the same time on finding other treatments that heal faster and are more effective for that type of illness.

El editorial de cierto periódico decía hace poco que una de cada diez personas en este país ha padecido alguna vez en su vida de demencia o de algún trastorno mental. Y aseguraba el comentarista que el 48 por ciento de la camas en los hospitales las ocupan personas con trastornos mentales. También consideraba que los trastornos mentales van en aumento con el correr del tiempo y el incremento de la civilización. Es por eso, según las palabras del editorialista, que se debe hacer más énfasis en el terapia intensiva y al mismo tiempo deben buscarse otros medio de curación que sean más rápidos y efectivos contra este tipo de enfermedad.

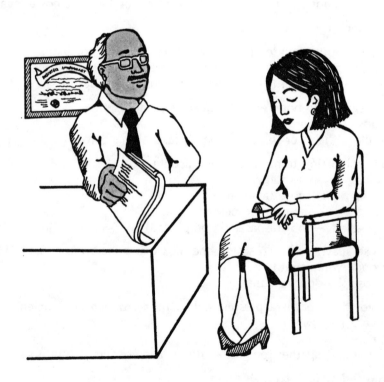

ADDITIONAL INFORMATION — INFORMACION ADICIONAL

1. Reasons for some nervous breakdowns — Motivos que ocasionan trastornos nerviosos

accidentes	— accidents
chascos de la vida	— unexpected setbacks
chismes	— gossip
decepciones	— deceptions
divorcio	— divorce
fracasos amorosos	— disappointments in love
fracasos en los estudios	— failure at school
fracasos en los negocios	— failure in business
guerras	— wars
incompatibilidad	— incompatibility
inseguridad en la bolsa	— stock market fluctuations
muerte de amistades	— death of friends
muerte de animales favoritos	— death of pets
muerte de familiares	— death of relatives
problemas de salud	— health problems
problemas familiares	— family problems
problemas financieros	— money problems
pesares	— sorrows
traición o abandono	— treachery or abandonment

2. Spanish last names — Apellidos ingleses

Abadía	Marulanda	Ferguson	Fuller
Colón	Navarro	Field	George
de la Rosa	Pantoja	Fillman	Gibson
Gallegos	Reina	Fisher	Glass
Guillén	Rivera	Fletcher	Goodwin
Gullón	Romero	Ford	Graham
Gutiérrez	Sepúlveda		
Manotas	Solís		
Martínez	Yepes		

3. Useful expressions — Expresiones útiles

Las preocupaciones pueden arruinar su vida	— Worries can ruin your life.
Haga una cita con la recepcionista	— Make an appointment with the receptionist.
La locura puede no ser hereditaria	— Insanity may not be hereditary.
La salud mental es muy importante	— Mental health is very important.
El siquiatra es una persona muy competente	— The psychiatrist is very competent person.
Cada día aumenta el número de suicidios	— Every day the number of suicides increases.
Descanse mucho y desaparecerá su ansiedad	— Rest a lot and your anxiety will disappear.
¡Cuidado con el nuevo paciente: sufre de demencia!	— Be careful with the new patient: He is suffering from insanity.
Usted debe abandonar sus pensamientos deprimentes	— You should forget about your depressing thoughts.

4. Idiomatic expressions — Expresiones idiomáticas

A lo lejos	— in the distance
¡Con razón!	— no wonder!
tal para cual	— two of a kind
volver en sí	— to recover one's senses
a tontas y a locas	— thoughtlessly, senselessly
agarrarlo con las manos en la masa	— to catch someone with the goods or with his hand in the cookie jar
creerse una gran cosa	— to consider oneself to be very important

5. Request for voluntary admission and authorization for treatment at St. Helena Hospital and Health Center.

The undersigned hereby requests admission to St. Helena Hospital and Health Center Neuro-Psychiatric Unit and consents to such care and treatment as is ordered by the undersigned's attending physician or his associates.

If my request is granted, I agree to conform to all rules and regulations and to give seventy-two hours notice in writing before leaving against medical advice. In the event of discharge against medical advice, I agree to wait until responsible relatives call for me.

If it is deemed by my physician or St. Helena Hospital and Health Center staff that my condition is not treatable here, I will accept discharge or transfer to another hospital.

I understand that any patient bringing alcoholic beverages and/or any dangerous drugs into the Mental Health Unit will be subject to immediate discharge.

I understand that the hospital may deem it necessary to search my person, my possessions and my hospital room for items which it considers dangerous to my safety and welfare or to the safety and welfare of other patients and hospital employees. I hereby consent to any such search of my person, my possessions and my hospital room which may be made by any hospital employee and release the hospital and its employees from any liability or other responsibility for the consequences of such a search.

I understand that it is the policy of this hospital to permit the maximum amount of freedom of action commensurate with my condition as an important factor in my treatment program. This freedom of action may lead to possible self-injury and I release the hospital, its employees and agents, as well as my attending physician or his associates, from any and all responsibility in case such freedom leads to injury.

5. Petición voluntaria de admisión y autorización de tratamiento en el Centro de Salud del Hospital St. Helena.

El que abajo firma solicita admisión al St. Helena Hospital and Health Center en la Unidad de Neurosiquiatría y autoriza el cuidado o tratamiento que ordenen el doctor o asociados que firman abajo.

Si se acepta mi petición, prometo estar de acuerdo con todas las leyes y reglamentos y presentaré un aviso por escrito setenta y dos horas antes de abandonar el hospital, si es que lo hago en contra del consejo médico. En caso de que salga contra el consejo médico, prometo esperar a que vengan a buscarme familiares responsables.

Si mi doctor o las autoridades del St. Helena Hospital and Health Center juzgan que mi condición no se puede tratar aquí, acepto que me hagan egresar o que me transfieran a otro hospital.

Tengo entendido que cualquier paciente que traiga bebidas alcohólicas y/o drogas peligrosas a la Unidad de Neurosiquiatría estará sujeto a la expulsión inmediata.

Tengo entendido que el hospital puede juzgar necesaria la requisa en mi persona, de mis posesiones y del cuarto donde esté, por cosas que se consideren peligrosas con relación a mi beneficio y seguridad y el beneficio y seguridad de otros pacientes y empleados del hospital. Por lo tanto consiento en cualquier requisa en mi persona, mis posesiones y el cuarto donde esté, la cual puede ser hecha por cualquier empleado del hospital y de esta manera eximo al hospital y a los empleados de cualquiera obligación o responsabilidad que pueda ocasionar dicha requisa.

Entiendo que de acuerdo con la política del hospital se me permitirá el máximo de libertad proporcionadamente a mi condición como un factor importante del programa de mi tratamiento. Esta libertad de acción puede llevarme a sufrir alguna herida por culpa propia. Si esto sucede, eximo al hospital, a sus empleados y agentes, a los médicos y a sus asociados de ser responsables de lesión alguna que pueda ocasionarme tal libertad.

Patient's Signature — Firma del paciente _____

Responsible Relative's Signature — Firma de un familiar responsable _____

Attending Physician's Signature — Firma del doctor _____

Witness — Testigo _____

6. The nervous system — El sistema nervioso

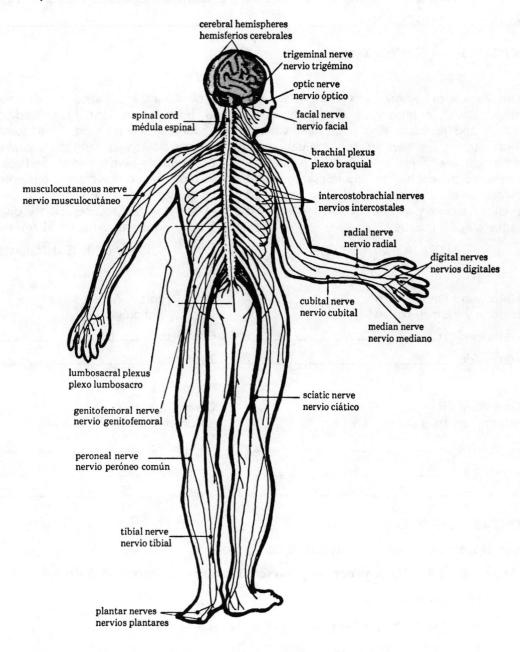

cerebral hemispheres
hemisferios cerebrales

trigeminal nerve
nervio trigémino

optic nerve
nervio óptico

spinal cord
médula espinal

facial nerve
nervio facial

brachial plexus
plexo braquial

musculocutaneous nerve
nervio musculocutáneo

intercostobrachial nerves
nervios intercostales

radial nerve
nervio radial

digital nerves
nervios digitales

cubital nerve
nervio cubital

median nerve
nervio mediano

lumbosacral plexus
plexo lumbosacro

sciatic nerve
nervio ciático

genitofemoral nerve
nervio genitofemoral

peroneal nerve
nervio peróneo común

tibial nerve
nervio tibial

plantar nerves
nervios plantares

BILINGUAL PROJECT — PROYECTO BILINGUE

TRANSCRIPTION — TRANSCRIPCION

Complete the following report along with the completed transcription. (See pp. 107-108).

Prepare la siguiente transcripción y termine los informes adjuntos. (Vea pág. 107-108).

NAME — NOMBRE: _____

ADDRESS — DIRECCION: _____

SITUATION — SITUACION: _____

This 28 year-old woman was admitted to the hospital with a history of abdominal complaints and jaundice. She underwent various X-ray studies as part of the evaluation to determine her illness. A consultant was asked to see the patient and to help in diagnosis and management. Her time in the hospital and eventual recovery and disposition are outlined in the clinical resumé.

Esta señora de 28 años de edad fue admitida al hosital con una historia de problemas abdominales e ictericia. Se le tomaron varias radiografías como parte de la evaluación para determinar su enfermedad. Se trajo a un consultante para que viera a la paciente y ayudara en el diagnóstico y los cuidados. Su estadía en el hospital y su recuperación y disposición se hallan esquematizados en el resumen clínico.

SEQUENCE OF REPORTS   —   ORDEN DE LOS INFORMES

A—1   A—2

History and Physical Exam   X-ray Report
Historia y examen físico   Informe radiológico

Completed _____   Completed _____

Terminado _____   Terminado _____

A—3   A—4

Consultant's Report   Clinical Resumé
Informe del consultante   Resumen clínico

Completed _____   Completed _____

Terminado _____   Terminado _____

EXERCISES — EJERCICIOS

(Students learning Spanish — Estudiantes de español)

A. Change the following sentences from present indicative to present subjunctive.

1. Los pacientes saludan ....

2. Los anestesiólogos hacen ....

3. El farmacéutico y su hijo trabajan ....

4. El siquiatra ayuda ....

5. El cirujano opera ....

B. Write six sentences using the imperative form.

1. ....   4. ....
2. ....   5. ....
3. ....   6. ....

C. Write a short composition describing the importance of the Neuro-Psychiatric unit.

....
....
....
....
....

D. Make a list (in Spanish) of the main causes of insanity.

....
....
....

E. Answer in Spanish.

1. ¿Cómo debe tratarse a una persona que intenta suicidarse? ....
....

2. ¿Cómo puede curarse la esquizofrenia? ....

3. ¿Por qué son tan solicitados los siquiatras? ....

4. ¿Por qué hay tantas personas con trastornos mentales? ....
....

5. ¿Qué puede hacerse con un loco que tiene tendencias criminales? ....
....

F. Translate into Spanish.

1. My neighbor tried to commit suicide. ....

2. There are many insane people at the Hospital for the Insane. ....

3. The psychiatrist is a medical doctor. ....

4. There is a neuropsychiatric unit in the hospital. ....

5. I work in the maternity ward. ....

EJERCICIOS — EXERCISES

(Para los estudiantes de inglés — Students learning English)

A. Escriba cinco mandatos en forma afirmativa y luego póngalos en forma negativa.

1. ....
2. ....
3. ....
4. ....
5. ....

B. Traduzca las siguientes oraciones al inglés.

1. Deme un remedio, por favor. ....
2. Ven y siéntate conmigo. ....
3. Vamos a comer en la cafetería. ....
4. Búsquelo en el diccionario. ....
5. Se prohibe pescar en el lago. ....

C. Redacte seis oraciones con palabras indefinidas.

1. ....   4. ....
2. ....   5. ....
3. ....   6. ....

D. Conteste en inglés.

1. Where is the Hospital for the Insane? ....
2. How do you treat a person who has suicidal tendencies? ....
3. Who is the psychiatrist? ....
4. Is there a neuropsychiatric unit in the hospital where you work? ....
5. What do you do on your days off? ....

E. Traduzca al inglés.

1. Yo conozco a una persona que tiene problemas mentales. ....
2. El manicomio está abierto al público los domingos. ....
3. El profesor será operado la semana próxima. ....
4. Buscamos a una secretaria bilingüe. ....
5. ¿Cuál es su problema principal? ....

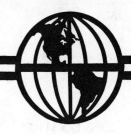

MAJOR ILLNESSES
ENFERMEDADES GRAVES

VOCABULARY — VOCABULARIO

A. Medical — Médico

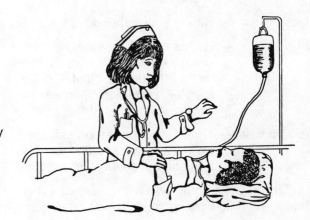

andador	— walker
artritis	— arthritis
cojo	— lame
defecto congénito	— birth defect
distrofia muscular	— muscular dystrophy
enfermedad genética	— genetic disease
epilepsia	— epilepsy
esclerosis múltiple	— multiple sclerosis
fibrosis quística	— cystic fibrosis
gangrena	— gangrene
hemofilia	— hemophilia
jorobado	— hunchbacked
manco	— crippled in one hand or arm, one-handed or one-armed
mongolismo, síndrome de Down	— mongolism, Down's syndrome
muleta	— crutch
silla de ruedas	— wheelchair
soportes	— braces
tartamudo	— stutterer
trauma	— trauma
tullido, inválido	— crippled

B. General

achaque	— sickliness	contemplar	— to watch
agilidad	— agility	débil	— weak
agonía	— anguish, death pangs	dinero	— money
		en seguida	— right away
alguna vez	— some time	espectador	— spectator
amputado	— amputated	entrada	— ticket
aplaudir	— to applaud	honor	— honor
atender	— to attend	padecer	— to suffer

pobreza	— poverty	tardar	— to be long
pueblo	— people	vejez	— old age

CONVERSATION — CONVERSACION

A. Jill Edwards takes her elderly father to the doctor for a regular check-up.

Jill   — Good morning, miss, I hope the doctor is not too busy today.

Receptionist — Busy as usual. But since you have an appointment he won't be long in attending to you.

Jill   — Thank you, miss.

Receptionist — How is your father doing?

Jill   — He has a good appetite, he sleeps well, but I've noticed that he's a little deafer, blinder, more crippled, more hunchbacked, and he stutters a little.

Receptionist — Those are illnesses of old age. Now I want you to fill out this form before seeing the doctor.

Jill fills out the form on which, among other things, the following information was requested:

Have you ever had:
 arteriosclerosis
 arthritis
 birth defects
 brain damage
 cancer
 cystic fibrosis
 diabetes
 epilepsy
 genetic illness
 heart trouble
 hemophilia
 hereditary defects
 kidney trouble
 meningitis
 mental illness
 mongolism
 multiple sclerosis
 muscular dystrophy
 nervous disturbances
 shock, trauma
 tuberculosis
 venereal diseases

Jill Edwards lleva a su anciano padre al doctor para un examen regular.

Buenos días, señorita, espero que el doctor no esté demasiado ocupado hoy.

Como siempre. Pero puesto que usted tiene una cita, él no tardará mucho en atenderla.

Gracias, señorita.

¿Cómo sigue su padre?

Tiene buen apetito, duerme bien, pero lo noto un poco más sordo, más ciego, más inválido, más jorobado y tartamudea un poco.

Esos son achaques de la vejez. Ahora quiero que llene este formulario antes de ver al doctor.

Jill llena el formulario en el cual, entre otras cosas, se pedía la siguiente información:

Ha padecido Ud. alguna vez de (del):
 arterioesclerosis
 artritis
 defectos de nacimiento
 lesiones del cerebro
 cáncer
 fibrosis quística
 diabetes
 epilepsia
 enfermedades genéticas
 corazón
 hemofilia
 defectos hereditarios
 los riñones
 meningitis
 enfermedades mentales
 mongolismo
 esclerosis múltiple
 distrofia muscular
 trastornos nerviosos
 un trauma síquico, shock
 tuberculosis
 enfermedades venéreas

GRAMMATICAL HINTS — APUNTES GRAMATICALES

A. Uses of the subjunctive in Spanish

1. The main difference between the indicative and the subjunctive is that the indicative states or denies a fact, while the subjunctive expresses a wish, desire, doubt, uncertainty or emotion as indicated by the verb in the main clause. The subjunctive in dependent clauses is normally introduced by the conjunction **que.**

2. Some of the most common uses of the subjunctive in dependent clauses are:

   a) After expressions of willing or forbidding.
      e.g. **Quiero** que el doctor venga temprano — I want the doctor to come early.
      Prohibimos que vayan a casa — We forbid them to go home.

   b) After expressions of doubt or fear.
      e.g. **Dudan** que lo opere — They doubt that he will operate on him.
      Temo que no se presenten — I am afraid that they won't show up.

   c) After expressions of joy or sorrow.
      e.g. **Siento** que no pueda salir — I'm sorry that she can't come out.
      Nos alegramos de que se esté mejorando — We are glad that he is getting better.

   d) After or with impersonal expressions except when they indicate certainty on the part of the speaker as to what is asserted.
      e.g. **Es probable** que la enfermera busque otro hospital —
      It's probable that the nurse will look for another hospital.
      Tal vez Juan venda la casa — Maybe John will sell the house.

   e) After a relative with an indefinite or negative antecedent.
      e.g. Buscamos **un técnico que** sea un buen radiólogo —
      We are looking for a technician who is a good X-ray man.

   f) After certain conjunctions when the verb denotes indefinite time or an action in the future.

cuando	— when	hasta que	— until
antes que	— before	luego que	— as soon as
aunque	— even if, although		

   e.g. Lo llevaré **cuando** venga el siquiatra.

   g) After certain conjunctions denoting purpose, proviso, concession, etc.
      e.g. Te digo esto **para que** (a fin de que) lo sepas —
      I'm telling you this so that (in order that) you'll know it.
      Puedes ir al cine **con tal de** (a condición de que) termines las tareas de la escuela —
      You can go to the movies provided you finish your homework.

3. The subjunctive is used in noun clauses after expressions already mentioned when the subject of the dependent clause is different from that of the principal clause. When the subject is the same then the infinitive is used.
   e.g. **Yo** quiero **ir** a la cafetería — I want to go to the cafeteria.
   Yo quiero que **Ud. vaya** a la cafetería — I want you to go to the cafeteria.

B. Verbos auxiliares en inglés

1. El verbo **can** (poder) tiene sólo dos tiempos, un modo (el condicional), dos formas solamente y no cambia de forma según el sujeto. En el presente es **can** (am, is, are, able, will be) y en el pretérito es **could.** No tiene infinitivo. **Can** o **Could** pueden significar:

a) Habilidad

   e.g. He **can** speak very well — puede hablar muy bien.

        He **couldn't** speak very well — no podía (no pudo) hablar muy bien.

b) Posibilidad

   e.g. She **can** lose her money — puede perder su dinero.

        She **could** lose her money — podría (pudiera) perder su dinero.

c) Permiso

   e.g. No one **can** see him today — nadie puede verlo hoy.

        No one **could** see him yesterday — nadie pudo verlo ayer.

2. Como **can** es un verbo defectivo el verbo **to be able to** lo reemplaza en los otros tiempos.

   e.g. The nurse won't **be able to** (can't) work tomorrow — la enfermera no podrá trabajar
                                                 mañana.

C. Más verbos auxiliares

1. **May** (poder), tal como el verbo **can,** es también defectivo y tiene sólo dos formas. **May** y **might** se usan para expresar:

a) Posibilidad o duda

   e.g. He **may** come back tonight — es posible que vuelva esta noche.

        She **might** arrive late — quizá llegue tarde.

b) Permiso

   e.g. **Might** I borrow your book? — me permite tomar prestado su libro?

        You **may** come in — Ud. puede entrar.

c) Propósito

   e.g. They are going every day so that they **may** (can) see the doctor —

        van cada día para ver si pueden ver al doctor.

2. Los tiempos del pasado son **may have** (de uso menos frecuente) y **might have.**

   e.g. He **may have** done that — puede que haya hecho eso.

        It **might have** been possible, but it doesn't matter —

        podría (podía) haber sido posible, pero ya no importa.

CONVERSATION — CONVERSACION (Cont.)

B. Santiago, Raul and Kent meet at work.   *Santiago, Raúl y Kent conversan en el trabajo.*

Santiago — Buenos días, muchachos, ¿cómo   *Good morning guys, how are you?*
          están?

Raúl   — Pues yo estoy bien, no sé cómo esté   *I am all right. I don't know how Kent may feel.*
          Kent.

Kent   — To tell you the truth, I don't feel   *Para decirles la verdad, no me siento bien.*
          completely well.

Santiago — ¿Qué te pasa?   *What's wrong with you?*

Raúl   — What's wrong with you?

Kent   — I feel weak; I have a headache, and   *Me siento débil; me duele la cabeza y la*
          my throat hurts.   *garganta.*

Raúl   — So you feel weak; you have **a**
          headache, and your throat hurts?

Santiago	— Dile que no trabaje hoy, que vaya a casa, que tome muchos jugos y que se acueste.	*Tell him that I hope he doesn't work today, that he should go home, drink a lot of juice and go to bed.*
Raúl	— Go home, drink a lot of juice and immediately go to bed.	
Kent	— I don't really want to go home because I have an aunt at home that is very sick.	*No quiero ir a casa porque ahí tengo a una tía que está muy enferma.*
Raúl	— No quiere ir a casa porque ahí tiene a una tía que está muy enferma.	
Santiago	— ¿Qué tiene?	*What's wrong with her?*
Raúl	— What's wrong with your aunt?	
Kent	— She has cancer.	*Tiene cáncer.*
Santiago	— ¿Por qué no la llevan al hospital?	*Why doesn't anyone take her to the hospital?*
Raúl	— Why doesn't anyone take her to the hospital?	
Kent	— The doctors say she can't be helped. She will die very soon.	*Los doctores dicen que no tiene remedio. Morirá muy pronto.*
Raúl	— No tiene remedio. Morirá muy pronto.	
Santiago	— Lo siento mucho.	*I am very sorry.*
Raúl	— I am very sorry.	

CULTURE — CULTURA

One of the most popular sports in Latin America, Europe, and many other parts of the world is soccer. Millions of spectators fill the stadiums every week, while others watch the games on television. In poor countries some people sacrifice their money in order to buy tickets to the stadium, so they can applaud their favorite team. In international games, very often the honor of a country is at stake, and on some occasions there have been unfortunate incidents that have caused the death of several people. This sport is very active and is played with great agility.

Uno de los deportes más populares de la América Latina, de Europa y de muchas otras partes del mundo es el fútbol (soccer). Millones de espectadores llenan los estadios cada semana, mientras que otros ven los partidos por televisión. En países pobres algunas personas sacrifican su dinero para comprar la entrada al estadio y así poder aplaudir a su equipo favorito. En partidos internacionales muchas veces se juega el honor de los pueblos y en algunas ocasiones ha habido incidentes lamentables que han causado la muerte de algunas personas. Este deporte es de gran acción y de mucha agilidad.

ADDITIONAL INFORMATION — INFORMACION ADICIONAL

1. Cardinal points — Puntos cardinales

norte	— north	este	— east
sur	— south	oeste	— west

2. The continents — Los continentes

Africa	— Africa	Europa	— Europe
América	— America	Oceanía	— Oceania (Australia, Indonesia and Adjacent Islands)
Asia	— Asia		

3. Geographical names — Nombres geográficos

Canal de la Mancha	— English Channel	Océano Artico	— Arctic Ocean
costa	— coast	Océano Atlántico	— Atlantic Ocean
frontera	— frontier	Océano Austral	— Antarctic Ocean
Mar Báltico	— Baltic Sea	Océano Indico	— Indian Ocean
Mar Mediterráneo	— Mediterranean Sea	Océano Pacífico	— Pacific Ocean
montaña	— mountain	país	— country
nación	— nation	río	— river

4. Spanish last names   Apellidos ingleses

Donato	Ortiz	Green	Hoover
Fernández	Peralta	Griffen	Hubbard
Hernández	Raíz	Hall	Jackson
Lince	Ramírez	Harris	Lamp
Martínez	Rodríguez	Hart	Lewis
Miranda	Sánchez	Hawkins	
Montoya	Sauza		
Nariño	Soza		

5. Useful expressions — Expresiones útiles

El paciente no debiera conocer el diagnóstico	— The patient shouldn't know his diagnosis.
Hay muchos casos de enfermedades incurables	— There are many cases of incurable diseases.
El paciente tiene un tumor maligno	— The patient has a malignant tumor.
El cáncer cuando está avanzado es incurable	— When cancer is too far advanced it is incurable.
Su caso es muy difícil, pero va a sanar	— Your case is very difficult, but you are going to recover.
Tenemos que operarlo inmediatamente	— We must operate on you immediately.
El enfermo tiene una terrible indigestión	— The patient has a very bad case of indigestion.
Tiene que comer más verduras	— You must eat more vegetables.
Algunos productos lácteos producen urticaria	— Some milk products cause hives.
El Departamento de Rehabilitación cuenta con un equipo muy moderno	— The Department of Rehabilitation has very modern equipment.
A pesar de todos los esfuerzos su cuerpo quedará afectado parcialmente	— In spite of all the effort, your body is going to be partially affected.

6. Idiomatic expressions — Expresiones idiomáticas

al cabo de	— at the end of	sudar la gota gorda	— to sweat profusely, to make intense efforts
al lado de	— at the side of, alongside of		
al poco rato de	— shortly after	tomarle el pelo a	— to kid someone
de suerte que	— so that	venir como pedir de boca	— to come (to happen) as if in answer to one's prayers
¿Qué hubo?, ¿Qué pasó?	— What happened?		
		vivir de gorra	— to be a parasite, to sponge
sin duda alguna	— without any doubt		
sobre todo	— especially	ya no	— no longer

7. Little poem — Pequeño poema

La paciencia todo lo alcanza.
Quien a Dios tiene
nada le falta:
sólo Dios basta.
(Santa Teresa de Jesús).

Patience achieves everything.
*He who has **God***
Needs nothing else:
God alone is enough.

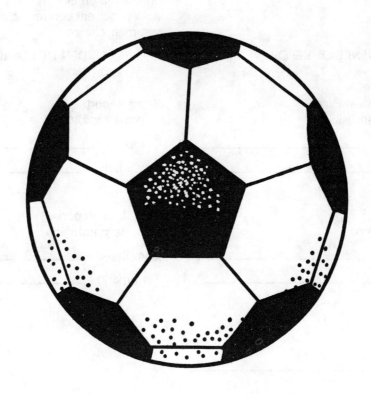

BILINGUAL PROJECT — PROYECTO BILINGUE

TRANSCRIPTION — TRANSCRIPTION

Complete the following report along with the completed trascription. (See pp. 107-108).

Prepare la siguiente transcripción y termine los informes adjuntos. (Vea pág. 107-108).

NAME — NOMBRE: _____

ADDRESS — DIRECCION: _____

SITUATION — SITUACION:

This 56 year-old woman with a lengthy history of prior medical problems was admitted seriously ill with symptoms of fever, weakness, headache, and cough. Her evaluation in addition to X-ray studies included an examination of her lower bowel during which an abnormal growth was removed surgically. The pathology report indicated this growth to be benign. Her hospital course and therapy are outlined in the clinical resumé.

Esta mujer de 56 años de edad y con una historia médica bien larga, que abarcaba muchos problemas anteriores, fue admitida al hospital en estado de gravedad con síntomas de fiebre, debilidad, dolores de cabeza y tos. Su evaluación, además de los estudios radiográficos, incluía un examen del intestino grueso (en el transcurso del cual se le extirpó quirúrgicamente un tumor). El informe patológico indicó que este tumor había resultado ser benigno. Su estadía en el hospital y la terapia que se le aplicó se encuentran esquematizados en el resumen clínico.

SEQUENCE OF REPORTS   —   ORDEN DE LOS INFORMES:

A—1   A—2

History and Physical Exam   X-ray Report
Historia y examen físico   Informe radiológico

Completed _____   Completed _____

Terminado _____   Terminado _____

A—3   A—4

Operative Record   Pathology Report
Informe quirúrgico   Informe patológico

Completed _____   Completed _____

Terminado _____   Terminado _____

A—5

Clinical Resumé
Resumen clínico

Completed _____

Terminado _____

EXERCISES — EJERCICIOS

(Students learning Spanish — Estudiantes de español)

A. Fill in the blanks with the correct form of the verb, either the infinitive or the subjunctive.

1. Ella espera (salir) _____ del hospital pronto.

2. El doctor espera que el enfermo (mejorarse) _____ pronto.

3. El siquiatra prefiere que los dementes (comer) _____ aquí.

4. Tal vez el médico (visitar) _____ a los pacientes hoy.

5. Mis familiares quieren que yo (ir) _____ a la clínica.

B. Fill in the blank in each of the following sentences by selecting the appropriate form given in parentheses to the right.

1. El cirujano _____ en esta ciudad. (vive, viva, vives)

2. Ella quiere que nosotros _____ la medicina. (compramos, compren, compremos)

3. El paciente viene _____ hospital. (al, el, de el)

4. Los enfermos _____ temprano. (se levantan, levantarse, levantan)

5. El doctor _____ operar hoy. (quiera, quiere, quieras).

C. Give the first person singular of the present subjunctive of the verbs given below.

1. beber . . . . 6. decir . . . .

2. hacer . . . . 7. tener . . . .

3. pasar . . . . 8. pedir . . . .

4. vivir . . . . 9. salir . . . .

5. esperar . . . . 10. pensar . . . .

D. Write six sentences with some of the idioms given in this lesson.

E. Before each of the following sentences place the phrase Espero que and make the necessary changes.

e.g. El enfermero viene — **Espero que** el enfermero venga.

1. No comen los pacientes. . . . .

2. El enfermo sale del hospital. . . . .

3. Los dementes no tienen problemas. . . . .

4. La farmacia está abierta. . . . .

5. La dietista sabe lo que está haciendo . . . .

F. Answer in Spanish.

1. ¿Cuáles son algunas de las enfermedades mayores? . . . .

2. ¿Qué papel desempeñan los neurólogos? . . . .

3. ¿Cuál es el mejor remedio para la gripe? . . . .

4. ¿Cuántas veces ha visitado usted el hospital este mes? . . . .

5. ¿Quién atiende la sección de registros médicos del hospital? . . . .

EJERCICIOS — EXERCISES

(Estudiantes de inglés — Students learning English)

A. Llene los espacios vacíos con alguna palabra apropiada en inglés que le dé sentido en la oración.

1. Please _____ us your telephone number.

2. Please _____ her your name and address.

3. Please _____ him the final score of the game.

4. Please _____ her your age and place of birth.

5. Please _____ me the name of your doctor.

B. Llene los espacios vacíos con la forma apropiada, ya sea can, could ó was able to. Si más de una forma es correcta, inclúyala.

1. The doctor finally _____ get in touch with the nurse.

2. We _____ visit all the hospitals.

3. Before the patient _____ play tennis.

4. After supper the technicians _____ work a little.

5. Last night he _____ sleep well.

C. Cambie las siguientes oraciones a formas negativas y después haga preguntas.
   e.g. They were able to do it. They weren't able to do it. Were they able to do it?

1. We were able to talk to him. ....
   ....

2. He says he can marry anyone he chooses. ....
   ....

3. The patient had been able to play tennis. ....
   ....

4. We think we can finish the work soon. ....
   ....

5. He said that I might borrow his car. ....
   ....

D. Conteste las siguientes preguntas con oraciones completas.

1. What's the most dangerous disease? ....

2. Where are you planning to go on your next trip? ....

3. What day of the week do you work less? ....

4. What's your wife's surname? ....

5. When are you going to be able to finish your education? ....

E. Haga una lista de las enfermedades más conocidas en la actualidad.

....

....

....

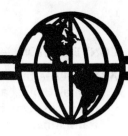

PUBLIC HEALTH
SALUD PUBLICA

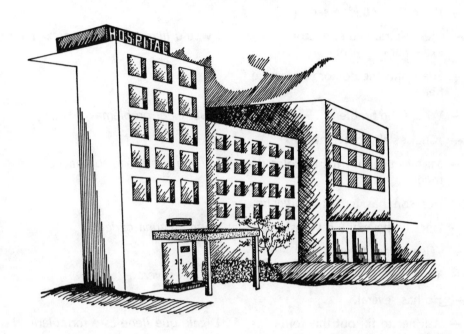

VOCABULARY — VOCABULARIO

A. Medical — Médico

agencias voluntarias	— voluntary agencies
camillero	— orderly
centros de aprendizaje	— learning centers
circulares	— circulars
consejo sobre la salud	— health counseling
deseos biológicos	— biological wants
empleos	— jobs, employment
hipoglicemia, dis- minución anormal de azúcar en la sangre	— hypoglycemia, abnormal decrease of sugar in the blood
informes anuales	— annual reports
instrucción o educación para la salud	— health education
preparación	— preparation
programas de clubes	— club programs
solicitud	— application
voluntarios	— volunteers

B. General

actualidad	— now, the present time
antes	— before
campaña	— campaign
cartas personales	— personal letters
carteles	— posters
desarrollo	— development
desempeñar	— to fulfill, carry out, perform
dueño	— owner
entidades	— institutions
función	— function
jefe de familia	— head of the family
papel	— role
precisamente	— precisely
propósitos	— purposes, intentions
publicidad	— publicity, advertising
reuniones	— meetings

CONVERSATION — CONVERSACION

A. Mrs. Olea takes her son Milton to the Mobil Dental Clinic, and the nurse asks her some questions. One of the other patients does the translating.

Mrs. Olea lleva a su hijo Milton a la Clínica Ambulante, y la enfermera le hace algunas preguntas. Uno de los pacientes hace la traducción.

Enfermera   — May we help you?

¿En qué podemos servirle?

Paciente   — ¿En qué le pueden servir?

Señora Olea — Me gustaría que el doctor examinara a mi hijo.

I would like the doctor to examine my son.

Paciente   — She wants the doctor to examine her son.

Enfermera   — What's the problem?

¿Cuál es el problema?

Paciente   — ¿Cuál es el problema?

Señora Olea — Mi hijo tiene un fuerte dolor de muelas.

My son has a bad toothache.

Paciente   — Her son has a bad toothache.

Enfermera   — Does he have any cavities?

¿Tiene alguna carie?

Paciente   — ¿Tiene alguna carie?

Señora Olea — Tiene varias.

He has several.

Paciente   — He has several.

Enfermera   — Ask her to fill out this form. It's bilingual.

Dígale que llene este formulario. Es bilingüe.

Name of the patient:
Nombre del paciente: _____

Address:
Dirección: _____

Date of birth:
Fecha de nacimiento: _____

Telephone (if any):
Teléfono (si tiene): _____

Father or guardian:
Padre o guardián: _____

Date:
Fecha: _____   Signature:
                                Firma: _____

GRAMMATICAL HINTS — APUNTES GRAMATICALES

A. Imperfect subjunctive in Spanish

1. The imperfect subjunctive of any verb is formed by dropping the ending (-**aron**) of the third person plural of the preterite tense and adding the proper ending: -**ara**, -**aras**, -**ara**, -**áramos**, -**aran**. A written accent is placed in the first person plural.

2. There are two interchangeable forms but we will study only one.

Hablar (hablaron)	**Comer** (comieron)	**Vivir** (vivieron)	**Ser** (fueron)
habl**ara**	com**iera**	viv**iera**	fuera
aras	**ieras**	**ieras**	eras
ara	**iera**	**iera**	era
áramos	**iéramos**	**iéramos**	**éramos**
aran	**ieran**	**ieran**	**eran**

3. Irregular verbs always follow the same pattern.

Infinitive		3rd Plu. Pret.	Imperf. Subj.
andar	— walk, go	anduvieron	anduviera
caer	— fall	cayeron	cayera
creer	— believe	creyeron	creyera
dar	— give	dieron	diera
decir	— say	dijeron	dijera
estar	— be	estuvieron	estuviera
haber	— have	hubieron	hubiera
hacer	— make, do	hicieron	hiciera
ir	— go	fueron	fuera
leer	— read	leyeron	leyera
oír	— hear, listen	oyeron	oyera
poder	— can	pudieron	pudiera
poner	— put, place	pusieron	pusiera
querer	— want	quisieron	quisiera
saber	— know	supieron	supiera
tener	— have	tuvieron	tuviera
traer	— bring	trajeron	trajera
venir	— come	vinieron	viniera
ver	— see	vieron	viera

B. El presente perfecto con <u>for</u> y <u>since</u> en inglés.

1. El presente perfecto a menudo se refiere a una acción que comenzó en el pasado y continúa desenvolviéndose en el tiempo presente. El período de tiempo puede extenderse de minutos a años.

2. **For** indica el tiempo que se ha demorado o durado la acción.
   e.g. He has lived (has been living) here for a year — hace un año que vive aquí (ha vivido aquí durante un año).

3. **Since** indica el comienzo de ese período de tiempo (a partir de qué momento):
   e.g. He has lived (has been living) here since 1959 — vive (ha vivido) aquí desde 1959.

CONVERSATION — CONVERSACION (Cont.)

B. Roger and Phil, two social workers, explain to a group of laborers the importance of owning their own homes. Roger took a double major while in college: Social Work and Spanish.

Roger y Phil, dos trabajadores sociales, le explican a un grupo de trabajadores la importancia de tener su casa propia. En la universidad Roger se especializó en dos ramas: Trabajo Social y Español.

Phil	— Mr. Sauza, since you are acquainted with this community, do you know more or less how many families own their own homes?	*Señor Sauza, ya que usted conoce esta comunidad, ¿sabe más o menos cuántas familias tienen casa propia?*
Roger	— ¿Sabe usted cuántas familias tienen casa propia?	
Sauza	— Muy pocas.	
Roger	— Very few.	
Phil	— How many of you would like to own your own home?	*¿A cuántos de entre ustedes les gustaría ser dueños de sus propias casas?*
Roger	— ¿A cuántos de entre ustedes les gustaría ser dueños de sus propias casas?	
(All raise their hands)		*(Todos levantan la mano.)*
Camacho	— Nos gustaría ser dueños de nuestras propias casas porque las rentas están por las nubes.	*We would like to own our homes because rents are sky-high.*
Roger	— Rents are sky-high.	
Gutiérrez	— Quince de nosotros vivimos en una casa de dos recámaras.	*Fifteen of us live in a two-bedroom house.*
Roger	— Fifteen people live in a two bedroom house.	
Martínez	— ¿Qué podemos hacer para tener nuestra propia casa?	*What can we do to own our homes?*
Roger	— They are wondering what they can do to own their homes?	
Phil	— We can look for federal aid.	*Podemos solicitar ayuda federal.*
Roger	— Podemos solicitar ayuda federal.	
Roger	— Nosotros les ayudaremos, pero tienen que trabajar unidos.	*We'll help you but you have to work together.*
Todos	— Así lo haremos.	*That's the way we'll do it.*

GRAMMATICAL HINTS — APUNTES GRAMATICALES (Cont.)

C. Sequence of tenses in the subjunctive mood in Spanish

1. A present or a future tense in the main clause is followed by the present subjunctive.

   e.g. **Quiero** que Ud. **vaya** — I want you to go.

   Haré lo que **pueda** — I'll do what I can.

2. A past or a conditional tense in the main clause is followed by the imperfect subjunctive.

   e.g. **Quería** que Ud. **fuera** — I wanted you to go.

   Si yo **fuera** rico, **tendría** otro coche — If I were rich, I'd have another car.

D. El condicional en inglés

1. El condicional en inglés se forma con el verbo auxiliar **would** más el infinitivo del verbo principal.

   e.g. I said that I **would go** — Dije que iría.

2. Se puede decir que el verdadero subjuntivo en inglés se expresa mediante la forma condicional, como ya lo habíamos explicado en lecciones anteriores.

   e.g. If I had money, I would take a long trip —

   Si tuviera dinero me iría de viaje por largo tiempo.

E. Hay palabras que pueden usarse para reemplazar toda una oración y de esta forma evitar cualquier repetición.

1. Too, so (también) se usan con ideas afirmativas.

   e.g. Peter works at the hospital. His brother works at the hospital.

   Esta expresión se puede cambiar de dos maneras: Peter works at the hospital and his brother works there too; o, Peter works at the hospital and so does his brother.

2. So puede identificar aquello por lo que se pregunta.

   e.g. Are you going to the hospital tonight? I think so.

3. Either, neither (tampoco) pueden emplearse para reemplazar oraciones negativas.

   e.g. I didn't study today. John didn't study today. Esta expresión se puede cambiar de dos maneras: I didn't study today and John didn't either; o, I didn't study today and neither did John.

COMMENTARY — COMENTARIO

Public health care plays an important role in society. That is why some federal and state agencies on the local level, together with regional and national medical and dental health associations, insurance companies, food products companies, and religious and educational groups, are concerned about the development of an open compaign in support of public health care. These agencies fulfill primarily the following functions:

1. administering first-aid
2. avoiding delinquency

La salud pública desempeña un papel muy importante en la sociedad. Es por eso que algunos departamentos locales, tanto estatales como federales, junto con algunas asociaciones regionales y nacionales de salud, ya sean sociedades médicas, dentales, compañías de seguros, de productos alimenticios, y entidades religiosas y educativas, se preocupan por el desarrollo de una campaña abierta en apoyo de la salud pública. Estas organizaciones desempeñan sobre todo las siguientes funciones:

— primeros auxilios
— cómo evitar la delincuencia

3. caring for the elderly	— cómo atender a las personas ancianas
4. child adoption	— adopciones
5. curing contagious diseases	— cómo atender a las enfermedades contagiosas
6. dental care	— cuidado dental
7. education in hygiene (health education)	— educación higiénica
8. family planning	— planificación familiar
9. keeping the family together	— cómo mantener la familia unida
10. medical education	— educación médica
11. pre-natal care	— cuidado pre-natal
12. preventive medicine	— medicina preventiva
13. post-natal care	— cuidado post-natal
14. raising children	— cómo educar al niño
15. sex education	— educación sexual
16. single mothers	— madres solteras
17. smoking, drug addiction, etc., and how to treat them	— cómo dejar de fumar y acabar con los vicios, etc.
18. stopping air pollution	— qué debe hacerse para prevenir la contaminación ambiental
19. taking care of a cold	— cómo atender un resfriado
20. teaching self-control	— educación sobre la temperancia
21. treating and preventing cancer	— cómo curar y prevenir el cáncer
22. understanding the housing problem	— educación sobre la vivienda

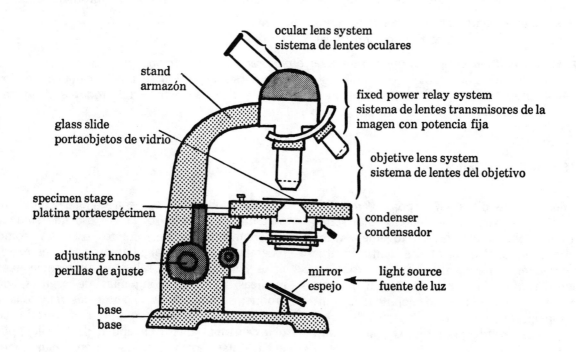

ADDITIONAL INFORMATION — INFORMACION ADICIONAL

1. Sightseeing — Lugares turísticos

acuario	— aquarium	lago	— lake
ayuntamiento	— town hall	mercado	— market
biblioteca	— library	mezquita	— mosque
castillo	— castle	monasterio	— monastery
catedral	— cathedral	monumento	— monument
convento	— convent	muelles	— docks
cueva	— cave	museo	— museum
cementerio	— cementery	palacio	— palace
estatua	— statue	parque	— park
estudios de		plaza de toros	— bull ring
videodifusión	— TV studios	teatro	— theater
exhibición	— exhibition	teatro de la ópera	— opera house
fábrica	— factory	torre	— tower
fortaleza	— fortress	tumba	— tomb
galería o museo de arte	— art gallery or museum	universidad	— university
iglesia	— church	viñedos	— vineydars
jardín zoológico	— zoo		
jardines	— gardens		

2. Spanish last names   Apellidos ingleses

Balboa	Manosalva	Logan	Paulson
Bastidas	Meléndez	Long	Rice
Bernal	Méndez	Martin	Smith
Castillo	Meza	Miller	Stevens
Duarte	Monsalve	Moore	Taylor
Flórez	Montalván	Morgan	Watts
Gómez	Niño	Morris	Williams
Guevara	Quintero		

3. Abbreviations — Abreviaturas

	English	Spanish
aa (ana)	of each an equal quantity	— de cada uno (a) la misma cantidad
ACS	American Cancer Society	— Sociedad Americana del Cáncer
AHA	American Hospital Assoc.	— Asociación Americana de Hospitales
AMA	American Medical Assoc.	— Asociación Médica Americana
ANA	American Nurses Association	— Asociación Americana de Enfermeras
APA	American Psychiatric Assoc.	— Asociación Americana de Siquiatras
A.R.D.	acute respiratory disease	— enfermedad respiratoria aguda
b.i.d.	twice a day	— dos veces al día
BM	bowel movement	— evacuación (de excrementos), corrección
BMR	basal metabolic rate	— rapidez del metabolismo basal
BP	blood pressure	— presión arterial
caps	capsule	— cápsula
CC	chief complaint	— síntoma principal
CHD	coronary heart disease	— enfermedad coronaria del corazón
CNS	central nervous system	— sistema nervioso central
CP	cerebral palsy	— perlesía cerebral

D.L.	danger list	— lista de enfermos graves
EST	electric shock therapy	— terapia de choque eléctrico
FH	family history	— historia de la familia
G.C.	gonorrhea	— gonorrea
Gyn.	gynecology	— ginecología
HEW	U.S. Health, Education and Welfare Department	— Departamento de Salubridad, Educación y Beneficencia de los Estados Unidos
HLR	heart-lung resuscitation	— resucitación de corazón y pulmón
H.S.	at bed time	— a la hora de dormir
I.C.U	intensive care unit	— unidad de cuidado intensivo
IQ	intelligence quotient	— cociente de inteligencia
IUD	Intrauterine contraceptive device	— pesario intrauterino
LHF	left heart failure	— falla del corazón (FL) izquierdo
L.M.P.	last menstrual period	— el período menstrual más reciente
M.D.	medical doctor	— doctor, médico
MH	marital history	— historia marital
MS	multiple sclerosis	— esclerosis múltiple
Non. Rep.	do not repeat	— no se repita
N.P.O.	nothing by mouth	— nada por la boca
o.d.	once a day	— una vez al día
P.A.	posterior-anterior	— posterior-anterior
p.c.	after meals	— después de las comidas
PH	past history	— historia pasada
P.I.D.	pelvic inflammatory disease	— enfermedad inflamatoria pelviana
P.R.N.	as needed	— cuando sea necesario
q.h.	every hour	— cada hora
q.i.d.	four times a day	— cuatro veces al día
q.2.h.	every two hours	— cada dos horas
RD	respiratory disease	— enfermedad respiratoria
RHF	right heart failure	— falla del corazón (FL) derecho
R.M.	respiratory movement	— movimiento respiratorio
sig.	directions	— instrucciones
s.o.s.	if necessary	— si es necesario
SR	stimulus-response	— estímulo-reacción
Stat.	immediately	— inmediatamente
T.B.	tuberculosis, "TB"	— tuberculosis
t.i.d.	three times a day	— tres veces al día
TPR	temperature, pulse and respiration	— temperatura, pulso y respiración
WHO	World Health Organization	— Organización Mundial de la Salud

4. Idiomatic expressions — Expresiones idiomáticas

¡Así es la vida!	— Such is life!
El paciente se recuperó notablemente	— The patient was as good as new.
hacérsele un nudo en la garganta	— to get a lump in one's throat
Los ancianos se recuperan más lentamente	— The elderly recover more slowly
perder la chaveta	— to lose one's mind
querer es poder	— Where there's a will, there's a way.
ser la mano derecha de uno	— to be someone's right-hand man.
sudar la gota gorda	— to make extreme efforts, "knock oneself out"
vivito y coleando	— alive and kicking.

5. Commands regarding law and order — Mandatos relacionados con la ley y el orden público

Apague el motor	— Stop your motor.
Cállese	— Shut up. Be quiet.
Deténgase, párese	— Stop
Entre en mi automóvil	— Get in my car.
Entregue sus armas	— Hand over your weapons.
Es la ley	— It's the law.
Espere aquí	— Wait here.
Está arrestado, detenido	— You are under arrest.
Firme aquí	— Sign here.
Hable más alto	— Speak louder.
Haga lo que le digo	— Do what I say.
Manos arriba, levante las manos	— Hands up. Raise your hands.
No corra	— Don't run.
No dispare	— Don't shoot.
No haga eso otra vez.	— Don't do that again.
No se mueva	— Don't move.
Póngase con la cara contra la pared	— Face the wall.
Póngase de pie. Párese	— Stand up. On your feet.
Quieto	— Freeze.
Salga	— Get out.
Siga caminando	— Keep moving.
Venga conmigo	— Come with me.

6. Useful expressions — Expresiones útiles

abuso de drogas	— drug abuse
beneficencia infantil	— child welfare
colaboración o columna médica periodística	— health column
condiciones de vida	— living conditions
desempleo	— unemployment
funciones de un profesor de medicina preventiva	— functions of a health educator
grupos minoritarios	— minority groups
La salud no es algo cómico	— Health is not a humorous matter.
los adultos pueden aprender	— adults can learn
madres solteras	— unmarried mothers
planificación familiar	— family planning
¿Qué es la instrucción para la salud (medicina preventiva)?	— What is health education?
relaciones humanas	— human relations
relaciones públicas concernientes a la instrucción para la salud	— public relations regarding health education
salud y beneficencia	— health and welfare

BILINGUAL PROJECT — PROYECTO BILINGUE

TRANSCRIPTION — TRANSCRIPCION

Complete the following report along with the completed transcription. (See pp. 107-108).

Prepare la siguiente transcripción y termine los informes adjuntos. (Vea pág. 107-108).

NAME — NOMBRE: _____

ADDRESS — DIRECCION: _____

SITUATION — SITUACION:

This 50 year old man had noted that over the three weeks prior to his admission to the hospital he had had an increase in the number of hypoglycemic reactions. He had a chronic cough which every morning was productive of whitish sputum. He had had some nighttime sweats, and at times he felt feverish. He was taken to the hospital where initial laboratory studies where done. His general condition deteriorated until he expired on the third hospital day. His hospital course and death are outlined in the clinical resumé.

Este señor de 50 años de edad había notado que durante las tres semanas anteriores a su admisión al hospital, había tenido un aumento en el número de reacciones hipoglicémicas. Tenía una tos crónica cada mañana que le producía un esputo blanquesino. Había tenido transpiraciones por las noches y a veces se sentía con fiebre. Fue llevado al hospital en donde se le hicieron inicialmente exámenes de laboratorio. Su condición general se deterioró hasta que expiró al tercer día de estar hospitalizado. Su estadía en el hospital y las causas de su muerte se hayan esquematizadas en el resumen clínico.

SEQUENCE OF REPORTS   —   ORDEN DE LOS INFORMES:

A—1   A—2

History and Physical Exam
Historia y examen físico

Laboratory Report
Informe de laboratorio

Completed _____   Completed _____
Terminado _____   Terminado _____

A—3

Clinical Resumé
Resumen clínico

Completed _____

Terminado _____

EXERCISES — EJERCICIOS

(Students learning Spanish — Estudiantes de español)

A. Rewrite the verbs in each sentence in the imperfect subjunctive.

1. Irá al doctor. _____

3. Yo como en la cafetería. _____

2. Tú operaste al paciente._____

4. Carlos y yo miramos la cirujía._____

5. El demente hizo mucho daño._____ 8. Esta tarea es muy fácil._____

6. El siquiatra leyó el mensaje. _____ 9. Luis trajo la cama. _____

7. La enferma no oye muy bien. _____ 10. El médico escribirá la receta._____

B. Change the verb in the main clause to the imperfect indicative and the one in the dependent clause to the imperfect subjunctive.
e.g. **Espero** que ella **vuelva** — **esperaba** que ella **volviera.**

1. El médico quiere que el paciente vaya al hospital. ....
....

2. Las enfermeras prefieren que los enfermos coman a tiempo. ....
....

3. Espero que mi hermana se mejore. ....

4. No crees que el demente salga del manicomio. ....

5. El anestesiólogo desea que el paciente pague la cuenta. ....
....

C. Write six conditional contrary-to-fact sentences.

1. .... 4. ....
2. .... 5. ....
3. .... 6. ....

D. Write a composition explaining the importance of health education.

....
....
....

E. Answer the following questions in complete Spanish sentences.

1. ¿Qué papel desempeñan los educadores de salud pública? ....

2. ¿Por qué es importante la planificación familiar? ....

3. ¿Por qué son perjudiciales los vicios? ....

4. ¿Qué papel desempañen las Clínicas Dentales Ambulantes? ....
....

5. ¿Por qué es de mucha utilidad la promoción de la educación sobre la salud pública?
....

F. Explain the importance of the Spanish language in the medical profession.

....

....

....

EJERCICIOS — EXERCISES

(Estudiantes de inglés — Students learning English)

A. Según la explicación de los apuntes gramaticales haga preguntas en el pasado usando el verbo que se da entre paréntesis. Luego dé dos respuestas, una con <u>for</u> y otra con <u>since</u> para indicar por cuánto tiempo y desde cuándo.

1. Dr. Simmons (work) for the hospital. ....

....

....

2. You (go) to the doctor recently. ....

....

....

3. The patient (be) sick. ....

....

....

4. The nurse (practice) her profession. ....

....

....

5. The pharmacist (work) for his parents ....

....

....

B. Traduzca al inglés.

1. Los hemos esperado por 20 minutos. ....

2. Hace cinco años que estudiamos inglés. ....

3. La medicina resultó ser excelente. ....

4. ¿Cómo está el paciente hoy? ....

5. Mañana me dan de alta. ....

C. En cada ejercicio combine las dos oraciones, de tal manera que formen una sola, evitando la repetición de ideas. (Vea los apuntes gramaticales).

1. You failed chemistry last year. He failed chemistry last year. ....

....

....

2. The doctor went home. The nurse went home. ....

....

....

3. The drugstore is open today. The school is open today. ....

....

....

4. They are intelligent. The student is intelligent. ....

....

....

5. We like medicines. He likes medicines. ....

....

....

D. Escriba seis oraciones condicionales contrarias a los hechos (hipotéticas).

1. ....   4. ....

2. ....   5. ....

3. ....   6. ....

E. Escriba una composición sobre la importancia de la salud pública.

....

....

....

F. Conteste en inglés.

1. Do you own your own home? ....

2. What do you think of social workers? ....

3. Why is learning English so important in professional life? . . . .
4. Who is your supervisor at work? . . . .
5. How much education do you have? . . . .

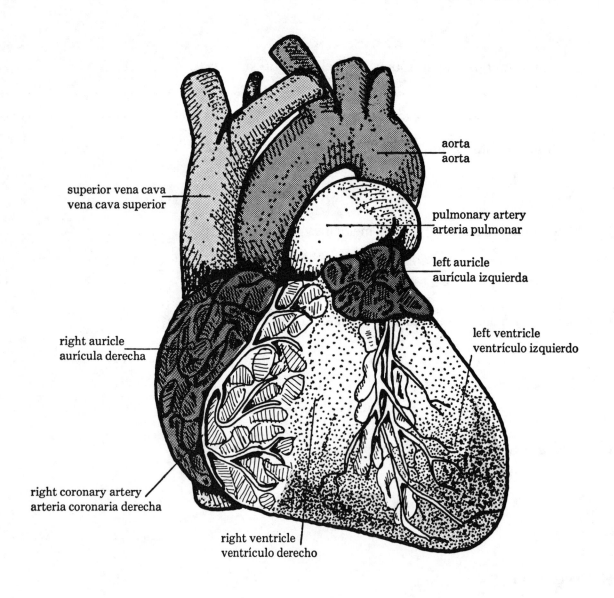

superior vena cava
vena cava superior

right auricle
aurícula derecha

right coronary artery
arteria coronaria derecha

right ventricle
ventrículo derecho

aorta
aorta

pulmonary artery
arteria pulmonar

left auricle
aurícula izquierda

left ventricle
ventrículo izquierdo

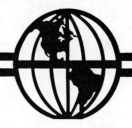

A

abdomen	—abdomen
aborto	—miscarriage
aborto provocado	—abortion
absceso	—abscess
abuso de drogas	—drug abuse
accidente automovilístico	—automobile accident
aceite de castor, de resina	—castor oil
ácido bórico	—boric acid
acidosis	—acidosis
acné	—acne
adicto a las drogas, drogadicto	—addicted to drugs, drug addict
admisiones	—admissions
adopciones	—adoptions
afecciones respiratorias	—respiratory disorders
afta, llaga	—sore, cold sore, mouth sore
agencias voluntarias	—voluntary agencies
agua destilada	—distilled water
aguarrás, trementina	—turpentine
agudo, grave	—acute, serious
aguja	—needle
aguja hueca	—hollow needle
ahogamiento	—drowning
ahogar	—to drown, stifle, choke, suffocate, asphyxiate
aislamiento	—isolation
al acostarse, a la hora de dormir	—on going to bed, at bedtime
albumina	—albumin
alcohol	—alcohol
alcoholismo	—alcoholism
alergia	—alergy
alérgico	—allergic
alfiler	—pin
algodón absorbente ó hidrófilo	—absorbent cotton
alimentación	—nutrition
alimentos sin refinar	—unrefined foods
almohadilla	—pad
alta tensión o presión arterial	—high blood pressure
alumbramiento o parto	—birth, delivery
alumbrar, parir, dar a luz	—to give birth
amalgama	—amalgam
amamantar, dar el pecho	—to breast-feed
ambulancia	—ambulance
amígdalas	—tonsils
amígdalas inflamadas	—inflamed, swollen tonsils
amoníaco	—ammonia
amputación	—amputation
amputar	—amputate
analgésico	—analgesic, pain reliever
análisis	—analysis
análisis de orina, urinálisis	—urinalysis
análisis de sangre	—blood test
andador	—walker
anemia	—anemia
anemia perniciosa	—pernicious anemia
anestesia	—anesthesia
anestesia local	—local anesthesia
anestesia total	—total anesthesia
anestésico	—anesthetic
anestesiólogo	—anesthesiologist
aneurisma cerebral	—cerebral aneurism
anfetaminas	—amphetamines
ansias matutinas	—morning sickness
ansiedad	—anxiety
antebrazo	—forearm
anteojos, espejuelos, gafas, lentes	—eyeglasses
antes de las comidas	—before meals
antiácido	—antacid
antibiótico	—antibiotic
anticoncepción	—contraception
anticoncepcional, anticonceptivo	—contraceptive
anticonceptivos	—contraceptives, contraception
antídoto para (contra) el envenenamiento	—antidote to poisoning
antiséptico	—antiseptic
antojo	—craving
aorta	—aorta
aparato ortopédico	—orthopedic brace or support
apatía	—apathy
apéndice (vermiforme)	—(vermiform) appendix
apendicitis	—appendicitis
apetito	—appetite
apoplejía, derrame, golpe de cerebro	—stroke, apoplexy
arteria	—artery
arteriosclerosis	—arteriosclerosis
arterosclerosis	—atherosclerosis
artritis	—arthritis
aseguradores	—insurers
asegurar	—to insure, assure
asfixia	—suffocation, choking
asilo de locos o dementes	—insane asylum

asistir a un parto
  como médico —to deliver a baby
asistir en calidad de
  médico, atender —to give medical help
aspirina —aspirin
astigmatismo —astigmatism
astillas —splinters
astringente —astringent
ataque —attack
ataque cardíaco —heart attack
atención médica —medical help
atención prenatal —prenatal care
atender —to give help, attend to
aturdimiento —bewilderment, grogginess
aturdir —to stun, daze
audiómetro, audióscopo —audiometer, earscope
aumentar de peso —to gain weight
aurícula derecha e
  izquierda —right and left auricle
axila, sobaco —armpit
azúcar —sugar

B

bacinilla, bacín —chamber pot
bajo(a) de azúcar —low sugar
baldado(a), tullido(a),
  inválido(a) —crippled, maimed, an
    invalid
banco, depósito de
  sangre —blood bank
baño —bath, bathroom
barbilla —chin
barbitúrico —barbiturate
báscula —scale (for weighing)
bata de operaciones —operating or
    surgical gown
bazo —spleen
bebé —baby
benigno(a) —benign
biceps —biceps muscle
bilis —bile
bisturí, escalpelo —surgical knife, scalpel
boca —mouth
bocio, coto, papera —goiter
bolsa amniótica —amnion, amniotic sac,
    bag of waters
bolsa de aguas,
  bolsa amniótica —bag of waters,
    amniotic sac
bolsa de hielo —ice bag, ice cap
bomba estomacal —stomach pump
boquilla —mouthpiece
botella —bottle
botica —drugstore, pharmacy
botiquín de primeros
  auxilios —first-aid kit
braguero —truss, brace
brazo —arm
bronquitis —bronchitis
bulla innecesaria —unnecessary fuss
    or noise

C

cabello, pelo —hair
cabeza —head
cada hora —every hour
cada dos horas —every two hours
cadera —hip
cafeína —caffeine
caída —fall
caja de Petri —Petri dish
calambres —cramps
calcañar, talón —heel bone, heel
calmante —tranquilizer
calorías —calories
callarse, guardar silencio —to be quiet,
    be still
calzar, rellenar,
  empastar, emplomar
  un diente —to fill a tooth
camilla —stretcher
camillero(a), asistente o
  ayudante médico(a) —medical orderly
camisa de fuerza —straitjacket
campanilla, úvula —uvula
canal auditivo —auditory canal
cáncer —cancer
cáncer del páncreas —cancer of the pancreas
capilares —capillaries
cápsula —capsule
caracol —cochlea
carbonizarse —to be scorched, burned
    to a crisp
cardiorespiratorio —heart-lung
caries —cavity in a tooth,
    tooth decay
carpo, muñeca —carpus or bones of
    the wrist, wrist
caspa —dandruff
cataratas —cataracts
catarro —heavy cold,
    influenza, grippe
caucho —natural rubber
cavidad bucal —mouth cavity
cavidad del ventrículo —ventricular cavity
cavidad dental —cavity in a tooth,
    tooth decay
cavidad uterina —uterine cavity
ceguera —blindness, loss of
    vision
cejas —eyebrows
células —cells
celulosa —cellulose
centro de aprendizaje —learning center
cepillo de dientes —toothbrush
cerebro —brain
cérvix, cuello del
  útero —cervix, neck of
    the uterus
choque —shock, collision
choque eléctrico
  electroshock —electric shock,
    electroshock
cianuro —cyanide
cicatriz —scar

ciclo gravídico	—pregnancy cycle	cordura, juicio sano	—sanity
ciencia médica	—medical science	corona	—crown
cintura	—waist	coronario	—coronary
circulación	—circulation	cortadura, corte, cortada	—cut, incision, slit
circulares	—circulars	cortarse	—to cut oneself, be or get cut
cirugía	—surgery, surgical operation	corva	—back of the knee
cirujano	—surgeon	costilla	—rib
cita, turno, compromiso	—appointment	costra	—scab
clavícula	—clavicle, collar bone	coyunturas, articulaciones	—joints
clínica	—clinic, hospital	coyunturas dolorosas, lastimadas	—sore, aching joints
clínica, etc., de reposo	—nursing home	cráneo	—cranium
cloro, decolorante	—chlorine, bleach	criatura	—baby
coagulación	—coagulation, clotting	crisis nerviosa	—nervous breakdown
coágulo de sangre	—blood clot	Cruz Azul, Escudo Azul	—Blue Cross, Blue Shield
cocaína	—cocaine	cuando sea necesario	—whenever needed
cociente o coeficiente de inteligencia	—IQ, intelligence quotient	cuarentena	—quarantine
codeína	—codeine	cuatro veces al día	—four times a day
codo	—elbow	cubrir, tapar	—to cover
cojo, tullido de una pierna	—lame	cuchillas, navajas para afeitar	—razor blades
colcha	—blanket	cucharada	—spoonful
colchón	—mattress	cucharadita	—teaspoonful
cólera	—cholera	cuello	—neck
colon	—colon	cuello del diente	—neck of the tooth
columna vertebral, espina dorsal, espinazo	—spinal column, spine	cuello torcido	—twisted neck
		cuentagotas	—medicine dropper
coma diabética	—diabetic coma	cuerpo	—body
coma, estado de coma	—coma, comatose state	cuidado de enfermero(a)	—nursing care
cómodo	—bedpan	cuidado dental	—dental, tooth care
comprimido, pastilla	—pill, tablet	cuidados intensivos	—intensive care
compañía aseguradora o de seguros	—insurance company	cuidado obstétrico	—obstetrical care
complejo de inferioridad	—inferiority complex	cuidado postnatal	—postnatal care
		cuidado prenatal	—prenatal care
compuesto químico, sustancia química	—chemical, chemical compound	curita	—Band Aid (trademark), small adhesive bandage
concepción	—conception	curar, sanar	—to cure, heal
concusión	—concussion		
condón, preservativo	—condom	**D**	
conducto lacrimal	—tear duct	dar a luz, alumbrar parir	—to give birth
conjuntiva	—conjunctiva	dar de alta	—to release from the hospital, consider cured
conjuntivitis	—conjunctivitis		
conminuto, fragmentado	—comminuted, fragmented	dar el pecho o la teta, amamantar	—to breast-feed
consejo médico o del doctor	—doctor's or medical advice	dar puntos	—to give stitches
consejos sobre la salud	—health counseling	darse prisa	—to hurry
consulta	—consultation	débil	—weak
consultorio del dentista	—dentist's office	decepciones	—deceptions
consultorio médico	—doctor's office	dedos de la mano, dedos del pie	—fingers, toes
conteo, recuento	—count, counting	defecto congénito	—birth or congenital defect
contra el consejo médico	—against medical advice		
contraceptivo(a)	—contraceptive	defectos de la vista	—visual defects
contraindicación de tratamiento	—inadvisability of treatment	defectos hereditarios	—hereditary defects
		deficiencia de hierro	—iron deficiency
contusión	—contusion	delgado(a)	—thin, slender
convulsión	—convulsion	delicado(a)	—medically serious
corazón	—heart	demencia, locura	—insanity, madness
cordón umbilical	—umbilical cord		

demencia senil	—senile dementia, loss of mental power due to age	divorcio	—divorce
		doctor, médico	—doctor, physician, **M.D.**
demente, loco(a)	—insane, crazy	doler	—to hurt, be painful
demerol	—demerol	dolor	—pain
dentadura	—set of teeth	dolor agudo	—sharp pain
dentadura postiza	—denture, false teeth	dolor de cabeza	—headache
dentífrico	—dentifrice	dolor de cuello, torticolis	—stiff neck, torticollis
dentina	—dentine	dolor de estómago	—stomach ache
depresión síquica	—psychic depression	dolor de muela	—toothache
depresión de postparto	—postpartum "blues"	dolor de oído	—earache
		dolores de parto	—labor pains
deprimido(a)	—depressed	dormir	—to sleep
derrame, golpe	—stroke	dosis	—dose
derrame de bilis	—bile flow	dosis excesiva	—overdose
desarrollo embrionario	—embryonic development, development of the embryo	dos veces al día	—twice a day
		droga	—drug
		drogadicción	—drug addiction
		drogadicto	—drug addict
desangramiento, pérdida de sangre	—bleeding	droguería	—pharmacy, drugstore
		ducha vaginal	—vaginal douche
desarrollo tardío (del habla)	—delayed (speech) development	duodeno	—duodenum
descongestionante	—decongestant	**E**	
desencanto de sí mismo	—loss of self-esteem	echar de menos, extrañar	—to miss, feel the need of
desengaño de amistad	—disappointment in friendship	eczema, eccema	—eczema
deseos biológicos	—biological needs	edema	—edema
deshidratación	—dehydration	educación médica	—medical instruction or education
desilusión	—disillusionment	educación o instrucción higiénica	—health instruction
desinfectante	—disinfectant	educación sexual	—sex education
desmayo	—fainting fit, spell of fainting	electrocardiograma	—electrocardiogram, EKG
desnutrido	—undernourished	electroencefalograma	—electroencephalogram
desnutrición	—undernourishment	electroshock	—electroshock
después de las comidas	—after meals	embarazada	—pregnant, with child
desvelo	—wakefulness	embarazo	—pregnancy
diabetes	—diabetes	embolia cerebral	—cerebral embolism
diafragma anticonceptivo	—contraceptive diaphragm	embrión	—embryo
		emergencia	—emergency
diapasón	—tuning fork	empleo	—employment, job
día por medio	—every other day	encías	—gums
diagnóstico	—diagnosis	encinta	—pregnant
diente molar, molar, muela	—molar, back tooth	enema, lavado del colón	—enema
dientes caninos	—canine teeth	enfermarse	—to become or get sick
dientes de leche	—baby or milk teeth	enfermedad o mal cerebrovascular	—cerebrovascular disease or illness
dientes incisivos	—incisors	enfermedad genética	—congenital disorder
dientes permanentes	—permanent or adult teeth	enfermedad hereditaria	—hereditary disease
		enfermedad nerviosa	—nervous disorder
dientes postizos	—false teeth	enfermedad siquiátrica	—psychiatric disorder
dieta	—diet	enfermedad venérea	—venereal disease
difteria	—diphtheria	enfermero(a)	—nurse
dilatación del cérvix, del cuello del útero	—cervical dilation	enfermo(a)	—patient, sick person, sick
dislocación de coyunturas, de articulaciones	—dislocation of joints	entablillar	—to put on a splint
		entre comidas	—between meals
disparo	—shot, discharge from a firearm	entregar	—deliver, hand over
distrofia muscular	—muscular dystrophy	envenenamiento, emponzoñamiento, intoxicación	—poisoning

enyesar	—to put on a plaster cast
epidemia	—epidemic
epilepsia	—epilepsy
epiléptico(a)	—epileptic
escaldadura	—scalding, burning
escalofríos	—chills
escalpelo, bisturí	—scalpel, surgical knife
escarlatina	—scarlet fever
esclerosis múltiple	—multiple sclerosis
esclerótico(a)	—sclerotic, hardened
escupidero	—spittoon, spit-bowl
esmalte	—enamel
esófago	—esophagus
espalda	—back
esparadrapo, tela o cinta adhesiva	—adhesive tape
espasmo	—spasm
especialista	—specialist
espejo dental, de dentista	—dental mirror
espejuelos, anteojos, gafas, lentes	—eyeglasses, glasses
esperma	—semen
espermatozoide	—spermatozoan, sperm cell
espina dorsal, espinazo, columna vertebral	—spinal column, spine, backbone
espinilla	—blackhead, shin, of the leg
espuma anticonceptiva	—contraceptive foam
esputo	—sputum, phlegm
esquizofrenia	—schizophrenia
estado civil	—marital status
estado de gestación, embarazo, gravidez, preñez	—state of pregnancy
esterilizar	—to esterilize
esternón	—sternum, breastbone
estetoscopio	—stethoscope
estilete	—probe
estimulante	—stimulant
estímulo: rección	—stimulus: response
estómago	—stomach
etiqueta, rótulo, marbete	—label
estreñimiento	—constipation
evacuación, defecación corrección	—bowel movement, BM
evitar contagio	—to avoid infection
examen de orina	—urinalysis
examen de sangre	—blood test
examen o reconocimiento físico	—physical examination
examen o prueba de Papanicolau	—Pap smear
excremento, materia fecal	—excrement, stool
extracción	—extraction, removal
extremidades	—extremities, members

F

factor Rh	—Rh factor
falla	—failure, deficiency
faja abdominal	—belly band, swathing bandage
falta de conocimiento	—unconsciousness
familiares	—family members
farmacéutico(a)	—pharmacist, pharmaceutical
farmacia	—pharmacy, drugstore
fatiga	—fatigue, tiredness
fecundación	—fecundation
fémur	—femur
feto	—fetus
fibrosis quística	—cystic fibrosis
fiebre	—fever
fiebre amarilla	—yellow fever
fiebre del heno	—hay fever
fiebre reumática	—rheumatic fever
fiebre tifoidea	—typhoid fever
flujo, secreción	—flow, flux, secretion
flujo blanco, leucorrea	—abnormal vaginal secretion, leucorrhea
flujo menstrual	—menstrual secretion or flow
flujo vaginal	—vaginal flow or secretion
forceps, tenazas de extracción	—forceps
formar	—to form
formulario, planilla	—form
fracaso amoroso	—disappointment in love
fracaso en los estudios	—failure at school
fractura	—fracture
fractura de la clavícula	—fractured or broken clavicle or collar bone
fractura de huesos	—bone fracture
frenillos dentales	—dental braces
frente	—forehead
frontal	—frontal, front

G

gangrena	—gangrene
garganta	—throat
gasa	—gauze
gastroenteritis	—gastroenteritis
gastrointestinal	—gastrointestinal
gelatina	—gelatine
genético	—genetic
ginecología	—gynecology
ginecólogo	—gynecologist
glándulas, endocrinas y exocrinas	—endocrine and exocrine glands
glándulas paratiroides	—parathyroid glands
golpe	—blow, stroke
golpe de cerebro derrame	—stroke
gonorrea, blenorragia	—gonorrhea

gordo(a)	—fat
gotas	—drops
grave, agudo	—serious, acute (illness)
gripe	—influenza, flu, grippe
guantes de goma	—rubber gloves
guardar silencio, callarse	—to remain silent or quiet

H

hambre canina	—acute hunger
hemofilia	—hemophilia
hemoglobina	—hemoglobin
hemorragia	—hemorrhage
hemorragia del sobreparto	—postpartum hemorrhage
hemorroides, almorranas	—hemorrhoides
hemostato	—hemostat
hepatitis	—hepatitis
herida	—wound, injury
herido de gravedad	—seriously wounded or injured
hernia	—hernia
hígado	—liver
hilo	—thread, string
hinchado	—swollen, swelled, bloated
hinchazón	—swelling, bloating
hipertensión, tensión arterial elevada	—hypertension, high blood pressure
hipo	—hiccup or hiccough
hipogástrico	—hypogastric
histeria	—hysteria
hisopo	—cotton swab
histerismo	—hysteria
historia familiar	—family history, record
historia marital	—marriage or marital history or record
historia pasada	—past history or record
hombro	—shoulder
hombros encorvados, cargado de espaldas	—slumped shoulders, round-shouldered
horas de consulta	—office hours
horas de visita	—visiting hours
hospital, clínica	—hospital
hueso	—bone

I

imperdible	—safety pin
impotencia	—impotence, impotency
incapacidad financiera	—inability to pay
incompatibilidad	—incompatibility
indigestión	—indigestion
inflamación	—inflammation, soreness
inflamatorio	—inflammatory, causing inflammation
influenza	—influenza, flu, grippe
informe anual	—annual report

inmunización	—immunization
insecticida	—insecticide
inseguridad financiera	—financial insecurity
insomnio	—insomnia
instalaciones de laboratorio	—laboratory facilities
instrucción o educación para la salud	—health education
instrucciones	—instructions, directions
instrumento	—instrument, tool
insulina	—insulin
internado(a)	—hospitalized, committed
intestino	—intestine, gut
intestino delgado	—small intestine
intestino grueso	—large intestine
intoxicación	—intoxication
inválido, baldado, tullido	—invalid, crippled maimed
investigación sobre el cáncer	—cancer research
inyección	—injection
iris	—iris (of the eye)
irritabilidad	—irritability

J

jabón	—soap
jaqueca, migrania	—migraine headache
jarabe para la tos	—cough syrup
jeringa, jeringuilla	—syringe, hypodermic needle
jorobado	—hunchbacked
juanete	—bunion
juicio sano, cordura	—sanity

L

labios	—lips
laboratorio	—laboratory
laboratorista	—laboratory technician
lactante	—lactating, producing milk
laminilla de vidrio	—glass slide
laparatomía	—laparatomy, incision in the abdomen
laringoscopio	—laryngoscope
latido del corazón	—heartbeat
latir, palpitar	—to beat (the heart)
latirismo	—lathyrism
lavamanos	—washbowl
laxante	—laxative
lengua	—tongue
lesión	—lesion
leucemia	—leukemia
ligadura de trompas	—tubal ligation
líquido	—liquid
líquido amniótico	—amniotic fluid
lista de enfermos graves	—critical list

llenar	—to fill, fill out, fill in
llorar	—to cry, weep
loción	—lotion, cream
loción contra insectos	—insect repellent
loción contra la quemadura del sol	—sunburn lotion
loción para broncear	—suntan lotion
loco(a)	—crazy, insane
LSD	—LSD
lunático(a)	—lunatic, insane, crazy
luxación de coyunturas	—dislocation of joints

M

madre primeriza o primípara	—mother for the first time, new mother
mal, enfermedad	—illness, disease, disorder
malaria	—malaria
mal cerebrovascular	—cerebrovascular disease
mal de rabia, rabia	—rabies
malestar	—discomfort, slight pain
maligno	—malignant
mama, pecho	—female mammary or milk gland, breast
manco(a)	—one-handed or one-armed
mandíbula	—jaw of man
manía depresiva	—manic depressive
manicomio, asilo de locos	—insane asylum, hospital for the insane
mano	—hand
máquina de afeitar	—safety razor
marbete, etiqueta, rótlulo	—label
mariguana	—marijuana
masticar	—to chew
martillo de percusión	—percussion hammer
máscara, mascarilla	—mask
media cucharada	—a half spoonful
medicamentos, medicinas, remedios	—medication, medicines, remedies
medicina, ciencia médica	—medicine or medical science
medicina preventiva	—preventive medicine
médico(a), doctor(a)	—physician, doctor
médico(a), cirujano(a)	—surgeon
médico de cabecera	—family doctor
medios de laboratorio	—laboratory facilities
medios o sistemas anticonceptivos	—contraceptive systems or devices
mejilla	—cheek
mellizos(as), gemelos(as)	—twins
meninges	—meninges (meninx)
meningitis	—meningitis
menopausia	—menopause
menstruación, regla	—menstruation, period

mentón	—chin
mesa de operaciones	—operating table
metabolismo basal	—basal metabolism
metadona	—methadone
método (anticonceptivo) del ritmo	—rhythm method (contraceptive)
microbiología	—microbiology
microscopio	—microscope
migrania, jaqueca	—migraine headache
molar, muela	—molar, back tooth
molde	—mold, pattern, form
molestias del embarazo	—discomforts of pregnancy
mongolismo	—mongolism, Down's syndrome
mononucleosis infecciosa	—infectious mononucleosis
mordedura (de perro)	—(dog) bite
moretón	—bruise
morfina	—morphine
movimiento	—movement
mucosa	—mucous membrane, mucosa
muerte	—death
muerte de familiares	—death in the family
muletas	—crutches
muñeca, carpo	—wrist, carpus or bones of the wrist
músculo	—muscle
músculo deltoide	—deltoid muscle
músculo doloroso	—sore muscle
músculo torcido	—twisted or pulled muscle
muslo	—thigh

N

nada por la boca	—nothing by mouth
nalgas	—buttocks, cheeks
narcóticos	—narcotics
nariz	—nose
nasal	—nasal
náuseas	—nausea
necesidad	—need, necessity
necesitar	—to need
nervio	—nerve
nervioso	—nervous, jittery
neuralgia	—neuralgia
neuritis ciática	—Sciatic neuritis
neurología	—neurology
neuromuscular	—neuromuscular
neurosis	—neurosis
niña del ojo, pupila	—pupil of the eye
no se repita	—no refill, no second time
nuca	—nape of the neck
nutrición	—nutrition

O

obesidad	—obesity, being overweight
objetos tragados	—swallowed objects

obstetra	—obstetrician
oftalmoscopio	—ophtalmoscope
oído	—hearing, ear
ojos	—eyes
ombligo	—belly button, navel
operación cesárea	—Caesarian section or birth
operación quirúrgica, cirugía	—surgical operation
orejas	—outer ears
órdenes médicas	—doctor's or physician's orders
órgano	—organ
orina, orinar	—urine, to urinate
oro	—gold
ovario	—ovary
óvulo	—ovum
oxígeno	—oxygen

P

paciente	—patient
pagar	—to pay
paladar	—palate
palangana	—portable washbasin or washbowl
palpitaciones anormales del corazón	—abnormal heartbeats, palpitations
palpitar, latir	—to beat (the heart)
paludismo	—malaria
páncreas	—pancreas
pan integral	—whole-grain bread
pantorrilla	—calf of the leg
paños esterilizados	—sterile cloths
paperas	—mumps
parálisis infantil, poliomielitis	—infantile paralysis, poliomielitis, polio
parientes	—relatives, relations
parir, alumbrar, dar a luz	—to give birth
párpado	—eyelid
partera	—midwife
parto, alumbramiento	—birth
parto o alumbramiento con fórceps (tenazas de extracción)	—forceps-assisted delivery
pasta de dientes, crema dental	—tooth paste
pastilla, píldora, comprimido, tableta	—pill, tablet
pastilla para dormir	—sleeping pill
pastilla para la tos	—cough drop
pastillas o tabletas anticonceptivas vaginales	—contraceptive vaginal tablets
paternidad responsable	—planned parenthood
pecho, pechos	—breast, chest, breasts
pedir ayuda, auxilio, socorro	—to ask for help
peligro de aborto	—danger of miscarriage
pelo, cabello	—hair
pene, miembro varonil	—penis, male organ
penicilina	—penicilin

pera de goma	—rubber bulb
pericardio	—pericardium
período menstrual, regla	—menstruation, monthly period
pesar	—to weigh
pescuezo	—neck of animals
pesario o dispositivo intrauterino (anticonceptivo)	—IUD, intrauterine (contraceptive) device or pessary
peso al nacer	—weight at birth
pestañas	—eyelashes
pezón	—nipple, teat
picadura (de insecto)	—bite, sting (of an insect)
picazón, sarna	—itch, itching, mange
pie	—foot
pie de atleta	—athlete's foot
piel	—skin
pies planos	—flat feet
píldora para adelgazar	—reducing pill
píldora, pastilla, etc., anticonceptiva	—birth-control pill
píldora, pastilla, comprimido, tableta	—pill, tablet
pinzas	—tweezers
piorrea	—pyorrhea
pisalengua	—tongue depressor
placenta	—placenta, afterbirth
planificación familiar	—family planning
planilla de inscripción	—registration form or blank
planilla, formulario, forma	—form, blank
plata	—silver
poliomielitis	—poliomyelitis, infantile paralysis, polio
política	—policy, politics
póliza de seguros	—insurance policy
pomada o ungüento de zinc	—zinc ointment
porcelana	—porcelain
potasio	—potassium
presentación de cabeza	—head presentation
presentación de nalgas	—breech presentation
problema abdominal	—abdominal problem
problemas familiares o personales	—family or personal problems
problemas financieros	—financial difficulties
profiláctico	—prophylactic
progesterona	—progesterone
programa diario	—daily schedule
programas de clubes	—club programs
programas de instrucción o educativos	—educational programs
próstata	—prostate
proteína	—protein
prueba de embarazo	—pregnancy test
prueba de Papanicolau	—Pap smear (Papanicolau's stain test)
puente, dentadura	—bridge

puffer, tampón —buffer
pulmón de hierrro —iron lung
pulmonía —pneumonía
pulmón, pulmonar —lung, pulmonary
pulpa (dentaria) —pulp of the tooth
pulso —pulse
puntos —stitches, sutures
pupila, niña del ojo —pupil of the eye
purgante, laxante —laxative

Q

quemaduras —burns
quemaduras del sol —sunburn
quijada —jaw of an animal
química —chemistry
quinina —quinine
quitar puntos —to remove
                stitches or sutures

R

rabadilla —coccyx
rabia, mal de rabia —rabies
radiografía —X-ray photograph
radiológico —radiological, of
                X-rays
raíz —root
rapidez del —basal metabolism
  metabolismo basal   rate
rayos X —X-rays
reaccion a la insulina —insulin reaction
receta o prescripción —prescription,
  médica   doctor's prescription
reconocimiento o
  examen médico —physical examination
recto —rectum
recuento o conteo de
  glóbulos rojos —blood count
recursos de laboratorio —laboratory facilities
régimen alimenticio,
  dieta —diet
registro o archivo
  médico —medical records
regla, período —menstrual period,
  menstrual, menstruación   menstruation
regulación de
  nacimientos —birth control
relaciones sexuales —sexual intercourse,
                sexual relations
remedio —remedy, medicine
reparar (tejidos) —to repair (tissues)
resfriado(a) —having a cold
respiración —breathing,
  respiratorio   respiratory
respiración artificial —artificial
                respiration
respirar —to breathe
resucitación —resuscitation
retardación, retardo
  o atraso mental —mental retardation
reumático —rheumatic
rico en proteínas —high-protein

riñón, renal —kidney
rodilla —knee
rubeóla —German measles
ruido innecesario —unnecessary noise

S

sacar la lengua —to stick out
                one's tongue
sala de emergencia —emergency ward
sala de espera —waiting room
sala de maternidad —maternity ward
sala de operaciones
  o de cirugía —operating room
sala de parto —delivery room
sala de recuperación —recovery room
salpullido —rash
salud mental —mental health
salvavidas —lifeguard, life
                preserver
sanar, curar —to heal, cure
sangrar —to bleed
sangre —blood
sano(a) —healthy
sarampión —measles
sarna, picazón —mange, itch, itching
seco(a) —dry
sedante para dormir —sedative for sleep
seguro de
  hospitalización —hospital insurance
seguro médico —medical or health
                insurance
seguro o seguridad
  social —social security
sentir —to feel
servicios prestados —services rendered
shock —shock
sicología, sicólogo —psychology,
                psychologist
sicosis —psychosis
sien —temple
siesta —nap
sífilis —syphylis
sietemesino(a) —seven-month baby
silla dental o de
  dentista —dentist's chair
silla de operaciones —operating chair
silla de ruedas —wheel chair
síndrome de Down, —Down's syndrome,
  mongolismo   mongolism
síntoma —symptom
sinusitis —sinusitis, sinus trouble
siquiatra, siquiatría —psychiatrist,
                psychiatry
sistema nervioso —nervous system
sistema nervioso central —central nervous
                system
síntoma principal —main symptom,
                principal complaint
sobaco, axila —armpit
sobreparto, puerperio —postpartum (period),
                post-deliverty
sociología —sociology

sodio —sodium
sofocation, asfixia —choking, suffocation, asphyxiation
solicitud —application (form)
solución antiséptica —antiseptic solution
solvente —solvent
sonda —probe, sound
soporífero —soporific, sleep-inducing drug
soportes —braces, supports
sordera —deafness
sordomudo(a) —deaf-mute
sudor, transpiración —sweat, perspiration
sulfato de calcio —calcium sulphate
supervisor(a) —supervisor
suplementos minerales —mineral supplements
supositorio —suppository
sustancia química compuesto químico —chemical compound
sutura, suturar —suture, to suture, stitch

T

tableta, pastilla, píldora, comprimido —tablet, pill
tablilla —splint
talón, calcañar —heel, heel bone
tapar —to cover, plug
tapón quirúrgico —surgical plug
tartamudo(a) —stutterer, stuttering
técnico de laboratorio, laboratorista —laboratory technician
tela o cinta adhesiva, esparadrapo —adhesive tape
temblor —tremor, trembling
temperatura —temperature
tenazas de extracción, forceps —forceps
tendón de Aquiles —Achilles tendon
tener el pelo castaño —to have dark or brown hair
tener exceso de peso —to be overweight
tener la lengua sucia —to have a coated tongue
tensión arterial alta o elevada, hipertensión —high blood pressure, hypertension
terapia, terapia intensiva —therapy, intensive therapy
termómetro —thermometer
testículos —testicles
testosterona —testosterone
tétano —tetanus
tetracloruro de carbono —carbon tetrachloride
tifus, tifo —typhus
tijeras —scissors, shears
timbre —bell
tiña, culebrilla —ringworm
tipo sanguíneo —blood type
tiroides, glándula tiroides —thyroid gland
tisis, tuberculosis —tuberculosis, TB
tobillo —ankle

tomar el pulso —to take someone's pulse
torcedura —twist, sprain
torniquete —tourniquet
tos, tos ferina o convulsiva —cough, whooping cough
toxemia —toxemia
trabajo de parto —labor
tracoma —tracoma
tranquilizante, sedante —tranquilizer sedative
trastorno nervioso —upset
trastorno ovárico o de los ovarios —disorder of the ovaries, ovarian disorder
tratamiento —treatment
trauma, traumatismo —trauma, injury
trementina, aguarrás —turpentine
tres veces al día —three times a day
triceps —triceps muscle
trillizos(as) —triplets
trombosis cerebral —cerebral thrombosis
trombosis coronaria —coronary thrombosis
trompa de Eustaquio —eustachian tube
trompa de Falopio —fallopian tube
tuberculosis, tisis —tuberculosis, TB
tubo de ensayo —test tube
tullido(a), baldado(a), inválido(a) —crippled, maimed, an invalid
turno, cita, compromiso —appointment

U

una vez al día —once a day
úlcera gástrica —gastric ulcer
ungüento —unguent, ointment
ungüeto o pomada de óxido de zinc —zinc oxide ointment
untar —to smear, daub, wipe on
unto —smear
unto, examen de Papanicolau —Pap smear
urgencia —urgency
urgente —urgent
urinálisis, análisis de orina —urinalysis
urticaria —hives, urticaria
útero —uterus
úvula, campanilla —uvula

V

vacío en el alma, depresión síquica —psychic depression
vacuna —vaccine
vacunación —vaccination
vacunar —to vaccinate
válvulas —valves
várices —varicose veins
vasectomía —vasectomy
vaselina —vaseline
vena —vein
venas pulmonares —pulmonary veins

venda de goma —rubber bandage
venda, vendaje —bandage
veneno —poison
venéreo(a) —venereal
ventrículo —ventricle
vértebra —vertebra
vértigo —dizziness, vertigo
vesícula biliar —gall bladder
veterinario(a) —veterinary, veterinarian
vida, vital —life, pertaining to life

viruela —smallpox
virus —virus
visita del médico —doctor's visit
vitamina —vitamin
volverse loco —to go crazy, insane
vómitos —vomiting, vomit

Y

yeso, enyesar —plaster cast, to put on or apply a cast
yodo —iodine

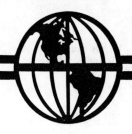

A

abdominal complaint	—problema abdominal
abnormal vaginal secretion, leucorrhea	—flujo blanco, leucorrea
abortion	—aborto provocado
abscess	—absceso
absorbent cotton	—algodón absorbente o hidrófilo
accident	—accidente
Achilles tendon	—tendón de Aquiles
aching joints	—coyunturas o articulaciones dolorosas o lastimadas
aching muscles	—músculos dolorosos
acidosis	—acidosis
acne	—acné
addicted to drugs, drug addict	—adicto(a) a las drogas, drogadicto(a)
adhesive tape	—esparadrapo, tela o cinta adhesiva
admissions	—admisiones
adult or permanent teeth	—dientes permanentes
albumin	—albúmina
alcohol	—alcohol
alcoholism	—alcoholismo
allergy, allergic	—alergia, alérgico(a)
amalgam	—amalgama
ambulance	—ambulancia
ammonia	—amoníaco
amnion, amniotic sac	—bolsa de aguas, bolsa amniótica
amniotic fluid	—fluído amniótico
amputate	—amputar
amputation	—amputación
analysis	—análisis
anemia	—anemia
anesthesia	—anestesia
anesthesiologist	—anestesiólogo
anesthetic	—anestésico
ankle	—tobillo
annual reports	—informes o reportes anuales
antibiotic	—antibiótico
antidote to poisoning	—antídoto para o contra el envenenamiento
antiseptic	—antiséptico(a)
anxiety	—ansiedad
aorta	—aorta
apathy	—apatía
appendicitis	—apendicitis
appendix (vermiform)	—apéndice (vermiforme)
appetite	—apetito
application	—aplicación, solicitud
apply or put on a (plaster) cast	—enyesar
appointment	—cita, turno, compromiso
arm	—brazo
armpit	—axila, sobaco
arteriosclerosis	—arteriosclerosis
atherosclerosis	—arterosclerosis
artery	—arteria
artificial respiration	—respiración artificial
arthritis	—artritis
asphyxiation	—asfixia, sofocación, ahogo
aspirin	—aspirina
at bedtime	—al acostarse, a la hora de dormir
athlete's foot	—pie de atleta
attack	—ataque
attend	—asistir como médico, atender, asistir
avoid infection	—evitar contagio

B

baby	—criatura, bebé, recién nacido
baby teeth	—dientes de leche
back	—espalda, respaldar
backbone, spinal column, spine	—columna vertebral, espina dorsal, espinazo
back of the knee	—corva
bag of waters, amniotic sac	—bolsa de aguas, bolsa amniótica
bandage	—venda, vendaje
Band-Aid (*trademark*), small adhesive bandage	—curita
barbiturate	—barbitúrico
basal metabolism	—metabolismo basal
bath, bathroom	—baño, cuarto de baño
beat	—latir, palpitar, golpear
be born	—nacer
become or get sick	—enfermarse
be or get cut	—cortarse
bedpan	—bacín, bacinilla, cómodo
bedsheets, sheets	—sábanas
bell	—timbre, campana
belly band, swathing bandage	—faja abdominal
benign	—benigno(a)

biceps muscle —músculo biceps
biological wants or —deseos o necesidades
  needs   biológicas
birth control —regulación de
  nacimientos
birth-control pill —píldora, pastilla,
  etc., anticonceptiva
birth —alumbramiento, parto
birth or congenital
  defect —defecto congénito
birth weight, weight
  at birth —peso al nacer
bite —mordedura (de perro),
  picadura (de insecto),
  mordisco
blackhead, shin of
  the leg —espinilla
bleach, chlorine —decolorante, cloro
bleed —sangrar
bleeding —desangramiento,
  pérdida de sangre
blindness, loss of —ceguera, pérdida
  sight   de la visión o vista
blood —sangre
blood bank —banco o depósito
  de sangre
blood pressure —presión arterial
blood test —análisis o examen
  de sangre
Blue Cross, —Cruz Azul,
  Blue Shield   Escudo Azul
body —cuerpo
bone —hueso
bone fracture —fractura o
  quebrantamiento
  de hueso
boric acid —ácido bórico
bottle, baby bottle —botella, biberón
bowel movement, BM —evacuación de
  excrementos,
  corrección
brain —cerebro
breast-feed —dar el pecho o la
  teta, dar de mamar,
  amamantar
breathe —respirar
breathing, respiration, —respiración,
  respiratory   respiratorio
breech presentation —presentación de
  nalgás
bridge, bridgework, —puente, dentadura
  denture   postiza
bronchitis —bronquitis
bruise —moretón
bunion —juanete
burn —quemar, quemadura
buttock, cheek —nalga

C

caffeine —cafeína
calcium sulphate —sulfato de calcio
calf of the leg —pantorrilla

calories —calorías
cancer —cáncer
cancer of the pancreas —cáncer del
  páncreas
cancer research —investigación
  del cáncer
canine teeth —dientes caninos
capillaries —capilares
capsule —cápsula
car or automobile —accidente
  accident   automovilístico
caries, cavity in a —carie, cavidad
  tooth   dental
carpus or bones of —carpo, huesos de la
  the wrist, wrist   muñeca, muñeca
cast, to put on
  a (plaster) —yeso, enyesar
cataracts —cataratas
cavity in a tooth, —cavidad dental,
  caries   carie
Caesarian birth or —parto u operación
  delivery   cesárea
cells —células
cellullose —celulosa
cerebral aneurism —aneurisma cerebral
cerebral embolism —embolia cerebral
cerebral thrombosis —trombosis cerebral
cerebrovascular disease —enfermedad
  cerebrovascular
cervical dilation —dilatación del
  cérvix o del cuello
  del útero
cervix, neck of the —cérvix, cuello del
  uterus   útero
cheek —mejilla, nalga
chemical —químico(a), sustancia
  o compuesto químico
chemistry —química
chest, breast —pecho, mama
chin —barbilla
choking —sofocación, sofoco,
  asfixia, ahogo
circular —circular
circulation —circulación
clavicle, collar bone —clavícula
clinic —clínica
club programs —programas de clubes
coagulated or
  clotted blood —sangre coagulada
coagulation —coagulación
clot of blood, blood
  clot —coágulo de sangre
coccyx —rabadilla
cochlea —caracol
cold —catarro, gripe,
  resfrío, resfriado
cold sore or
  similar sore —afta, llaga
colon —colon
coma, comatose state —coma, estado de
  coma
comminuted or —conminuto o
  fragmented   fragmentado

complication	—complicación
compress, hot compress	—compresa, fomentos
conception	—concepción
concussion	—concusión
condom	—condón, preservativo
congenital defect	—defecto congénito
conjunctiva	—conjuntiva
consider cured, to release from the hospital	—dar de alta
consultation	—consulta
contraceptive	—anticonceptivo(a), contraceptivo(a), anticoncepcional
contraception	—anticoncepción
contraceptive diaphragm	—diafragma anticonceptivo
contraceptive foam	—espuma anticonceptiva
contraceptive systems or devices	—sistemas o medios anticonceptivos
contraceptives, contraception	—anticonceptivos
constipation	—estreñimiento
convulsion	—convulsión
coronary thrombosis	—trombosis coronaria
cotton swab	—hisopo
count	—conteo, recuento
cover	—cubrir, tapar
cramps	—calambres
cranium	—cráneo
craving	—antojo, deseo intenso
crazy	—loco(a)
crippled, maimed	—baldado(a), inválido(a), tullido(a)
crippled in or a missing one hand or arm	—manco(a)
crown	—corona
crutches	—muletas
cry, weep	—llorar
cut	—cortadura, corte, cortada, cortar
cut oneself, to be or get cut	—cortarse
cystic fibrosis	—fibrosis cística

D

daily schedule	—programa diario
dandruff	—caspa
danger of miscarriage	—peligro de aborto
deaf-mute	—sordomudo(a)
deafness	—sordera
death	—muerte
death in the family	—muerte de familiares
deception	—decepción
delayed (speech) development	—desarrollo tardío (del habla)
deliver a baby	—asistir a un parto en calidad de médico

delivery	—alumbramiento
delivery room	—sala de parto
deltoid muscle	—músculo deltoide
demerol	—demerol
dental braces	—frenillos dentales
dental mirror	—espejo dental o de dentista
dentifrice	—dentífrico
dentine	—dentina
dentist's chair	—silla de dentista
dentist's office	—consultorio del dentista
denture, false teeth	—dentadura postiza, dientes postizos
depressed	—deprimido(a)
depression, psychic depression	—depresión, depresión síquica
diabetes	—diabetes
diet	—dieta, régimen alimenticio
disappointment	—desilusión, decepción, desengaño, contratiempo
disappointment in friendship	—desengaño de amistad
disappointment in love	—fracaso amoroso
discomfort	—malestar, dolor leve
discomforts of pregnancy	—molestias del embarazo
disillusion	—desilusión
disillusionment with oneself	—desencanto de sí mismo
dislocation of joints	—dislocación o luxación de articulaciones o coyunturas
divorce	—divorcio
dizzines	—vértigo
doctor, physician	—doctor(a), médico(a)
doctor's or medical advice	—consejo médico o del doctor
doctor's office	—consultorio médico
doctor's orders	—órdenes médicas, indicaciones del médico
doctor's prescription	—receta médica
doctor's visit	—visita del médico o del doctor
dose	—dosis
Down's syndrome, mongolism	—síndrome de Down, mongolismo
drops	—gotas
drown	—ahogarse en el agua u otro líquido
drowning	—ahogamiento
drug addict, drug addiction	—drogadicto, drogadicción
drugstore	—farmacia, droguería, botica
duodenum	—duodeno

E

earache	—dolor de oído
earscope, audiometer	—audiómetro, audióscopo
eczema	—eczema, eccema
educational programs	—programas de instrucción o educativos
elbow	—codo
electric shock, electroshock	—choque eléctrico, electroshock
electrocardiogram, EKG	—electrocardiograma
embryo	—embrión
emergency	—emergencia
emergency room	—sala de emergencias
employment, job	—empleo(s)
enamel	—esmalte
edema	—edema, excess water in tissues
embryonic development, development of the embryo	—desarrollo embrionario o del embrión
enema	—enema, lavado del colon
epilepsy	—epilepsia
epileptic	—epiléptico(a)
esophagus	—esófago
eustachian tube	—trompa de Eustaquio
every hour	—cada hora
every other day	—día por medio, un día sí otro no
every two hours	—cada dos horas
excrement, stool, feces	—excremento, materia fecal
extraction, removal	—extracción
extremities	—extremidades
eyebrows	—cejas
eyeglasses, glasses	—espejuelos, anteojos, gafas, lentes
eyelashes	—pestañas
eyelids	—párpados
eyes	—ojos

F

failure at school	—fracaso en los estudios
fainting fit, spell of fainting	—desmayo, pérdida de conocimiento
fallopian tube	—trompa de Falopio, oviducto de los mamíferos
family doctor	—médico de cabecera
family members	—familiares, miembros de una familia
family or personal problems	—problemas familiares o personales
family planning	—planificación familiar
fat	—gordo(a)
fatigue	—fatiga
fecundation	—fecundación

feel	—sentir, palpar
feeling of emptiness, psychic depression	—vacío en el alma, depresión síquica
female mammary or milk gland, breast	—mama, pecho
femur	—fémur
fetus	—feto
fever	—fiebre
fill a tooth	—rellenar, empastar, emplomar, calzar un diente
fill out	—llenar (un formulario o planilla), hacer aumentar de peso
financial insecurity	—inseguridad financiera
financial problems	—problemas financieros
fingers, toes	—dedos de la mano, dedos del pie
first-aid kit	—botiquín o equipo de primeros auxilios
flat feet	—pies planos
flow, flux, secretion	—flujo, secreción
flu, influenza	—influenza, catarro, gripe
foot	—pie
forceps	—forceps, tenazas de extracción
forceps-assisted delivery	—parto o alumbramiento con forceps
forearm	—antebrazo
forehead	—frente
form	—planilla, formulario, forma, formar
fracture	—fractura, quebrantamiento
frontal, front	—frontal
front teeth	—dientes incisivos

G

gall bladder	—vesícula biliar
gangrene	—gangrena
gastric ulcer	—úlcera gástrica
gastrointestinal	—gastrointestinal
gauze	—gasa
gelatine	—gelatina
genetic disease	—enfermedad genética
German measles	—rubeóla
give birth	—dar a luz, alumbrar, parir
give stitches	—dar puntadas o puntos
glands	—glándulas
go crazy, insane	—volverse loco
gold	—oro
gums	—encías
gynecologist	—ginecólogo
gynecology	—ginecología

H

hair	—pelo, cabello
hand	—mano
have a coated tongue	—tener la lengua sucia

hawking	—flema clara	incompatibility	—incompatibilidad
hay fever	—fiebre del heno	infantile paralysis,	—parálisis infantil,
head	—cabeza	polio	poliomielitis
head presentation	—presentación de cabeza	inferiority complex	—complejo de
heal	—curar, sanar		inferioridad
health counseling	—consejos sobre la	influenza, flu	—influenza, catarro,
	salud		gripe
health education	—instrucción o educación	injection	—inyección
	higiénica o para	inner ear	—oído
	la salud	insane	—demente, loco(a)
health insurance	—seguro médico	insane asylum,	—manicomio, asilo
healthy	—sano(a)	hospital for the	u hospital de
heart	—corazón	insane	locos o dementes
heart attack	—ataque cardíaco	insanity	—locura, demencia
heartbeat	—latido o palpitación	insect repellent	—loción contra
	del corazón		los insectos
heart-lung	—cardiorespiratorio	insomnia	—insomnio
heart palpitations	—palpitaciones	instrument	—instrumento
(abnormal)	(anormales) del corazón	insulin	—insulina
heatstroke, sunstroke	—insolación	insulin reaction	—reacción a la
heavy cold	—catarro, influenza		insulina
heel, heel bone	—talón, calcañar	insurance company	—compañía aseguradora
hemophilia	—hemofilia		o de seguros
hemoglobin	—hemoglobina	insurance policy	—póliza de seguros
hemorrhage	—hemorragia	insurance premium	—prima
hemorrhoids	—hemorroides, almorranas	insure	—asegurar
hereditary disease	—enfermedad	intensive care	—cuidados intensivos
	hereditaria	intensive therapy	—terapia intensiva
hiccup or hiccough	—hipo	intercourse (sexual)	
high blood pressure,	—tensión arterial alta	sexual relations	—relaciones sexuales
hypertension	o elevada,	iodine	—yodo
	hipertensión	IQ, inteligence	—cociente o
high-protein	—rico(a) en proteínas	quotient	coeficiente de
hip	—cadera		inteligencia
hives, urticaria	—urticaria	iris	—iris
hollow needle	—aguja hueca	iron deficiency	—deficiencia de
hurt	—doler, lastimar		hierro
hospital for the	—manicomio, asilo u	iron lung	—pulmón de hierro
insane	hospital para locos	irritability	—irritabilidad
	o dementes	isolation	—aislamiento
hospital insurance	—seguro de	itch, mange	—picazón, sarna
	hospitalización		
hospitalized	—internado(a)	**J**	
hunchbacked,	—jorobado(a),		
humpbacked	giboso(a)	jaw of an animal	—quijada
hypertension, high	—hipertensión, tensión	jaw of man	—mandíbula
blood pressure	arterial alta o	jobs	—empleos
	elevada	joints	—coyunturas,
hypodermic needle	—jeringa,		articulaciones
syringe	jeringuilla		
hypogastric	—hipogástrico(a)	**K**	
hypoglycemia	—hipoglicemia		
		knee	—rodilla
I			
		L	
illness, sickness	—enfermedad, mal		
immunization	—inmunización	label	—etiqueta, rótulo,
impotence	—impotencia		marbete
inability to pay	—incapacidad	labor	—trabajo de parto
	financiera	laboratory	—laboratorio
inadvisability of	—contraindicación	laboratory facilities	—medios,
treatment	de tratamiento		instalaciones, recursos
in between meals	—entre comidas		de laboratorio

laboratory technician —técnico de laboratorio,
                        laboratorista
labor pains   —dolores de parto
lactating   —lactante
lame   —cojo(a), tullido(a)
                        de una pierna
laparatomy   —laparatomía
large intestine   —intestino grueso
laxative   —laxante, purgante
learning center   —centro de aprendizaje
lesion   —lesión
leukemia   —leucemia
life   —vida
life guard, life
  preserver   —salvavidas
lips   —labios
liver   —hígado
local anesthesia   —anestesia local
loss of consciousness —pérdida de
                        conocimiento
lotion   —loción
low sugar   —bajo(a) de azúcar
lunatic   —lunático(a), loco(a)
lung, pulmonary   —pulmón, pulmonar

M

maimed, crippled   —baldado, inválido,
                        tullido
malaria   —malaria
malignant   —maligno
malnutrition   —desnutrición
mange, itch   —sarna, picazón
manic depression   —manía depresiva
mask   —máscara, mascarilla
maternity ward   —sala de maternidad
medical advice   —consejo médico
medical science   —ciencia médica
medically serious   —delicado(a), grave
medicine   —medicina, medicamento,
                        remedio
medicine dropper   —cuentagotas
meningitis   —meningitis
menstrual period,   —regla, período
  menstruation   menstrual,
                        menstruación
menstrual secretion
  or flow   —flujo menstrual
mental retardation   —retardación, retardo,
                        retraso mental
metabolism   —metabolismo
microscope   —microscopio
midwife   —partera
migraine   —migrania, jaqueca
mineral supplements   —suplementos minerales
miscarriage   —aborto, mal parto
miss   —echar de menos,
                        extrañar, no acertar
molar   —diente molar, molar
                        muela
mongolism, Down's   —mongolismo,
  syndrome   síndrome de Down
morning sickness   —ansias matutinas

morphine   —morfina
mouth   —boca
mouth cavity   —cavidad bucal
mucous membrane   —mucosa
multiple birth   —alumbramiento o
                        parto múltiple
multiple sclerosis   —esclerosis múltiple
mumps   —paperas
muscles   —músculos
muscular dystrophy   —distrofia muscular

N

nap   —siesta
nape of the neck   —nuca
nasal   —nasal
navel   —ombligo
neck of man   —cuello
neck of animals   —pescuezo
neck of a tooth   —cuello del diente
need   —necesitar, necesidad
needle   —aguja
nerve   —nervio
nervous   —nervioso(a)
nervous system   —sistema nervioso
neurological disorder —enfermedades
                        nerviosas
neurology   —neurología
neuromuscular   —neuromuscular
nipple, teat   —pezón
nothing by mouth   —nada por la boca
nurse   —enfermero(a)
nursing care   —cuidado de
                        enfermero(a)
nursing home   —clínica, etc. de
                        reposo
nutrition   —nutrición, alimentación
nutritional   —alimenticio

O

obesity   —obesidad
obstetrician   —obstetra
one-handed or one-
  armed   —manco(a)
operating chair   —silla de operaciones
operating room   —sala de operaciones
                        o de cirugía
operating table   —mesa de operaciones
                        o de cirugía
ophthalmoscope   —oftalmoscopio
orderly   —camillero(a),
                        asistente o
                        ayudante médico
organ   —órgano
orthopedic brace or
  support   —aparato ortopédico
outer ears   —orejas
ovarian disorders,
  disorders of the
  ovaries   —trastornos ováricos
                        o de los ovarios
ovary   —ovario
overdose   —dosis excesiva

ovum	—óvulo	premarital	—prenupcial
oxygen	—oxígeno	premature birth	—alumbramiento o parto prematuro
P		prenatal care	—atención prenatal
		preparation	—preparación
pain	—dolor	prescription	—receta, prescripción
palate	—paladar	premium	—prima
pancreas	—páncreas	probe, sound	—sonda
Pap smear (Papanicolau's stain test)	—prueba de Papanicolau	psychiatric disorder	—enfermedad siquiátrica
parathyroid glands	—glándulas paratiroides	psychiatrist	—siquiatra
		psychiatry	—siquiatría
patient, sick person	—paciente, enfermo(a)	psychologist	—sicólogo
		psychology	—sicología
pay	—pagar	psychic depression, depression	—depresión síquica, depresión
penicilin	—penicilina	psychosis	—sicosis
penis, male organ	—pene, miembro varonil	pulmonary veins	—venas pulmonares
pericardium	—pericardio	pulp (of a tooth)	—pulpa (dentaria)
permanent or adult teeth	—dientes permanentes	pulse	—pulso
		pupil of the eye	—pupila, niña del ojo
pernicious anemia	—anemia perniciosa	purgative	—purgante, laxante
persistent vomiting	—vómitos persistentes	put on a plaster cast	—enyesar
pharmaceutic, pharmacist	—farmacéutico(a)	put on a splint	—entablillar
pharmacy	—farmacia, droguería, botica	pyorrea	—piorrea
physical examination	—examen o reconocimiento físico	**Q**	
		quarantine	—cuarentena
physician, doctor	—médico(a), doctor(a)	quinine	—quinina
pill	—píldora, pastilla, comprimido, tableta	**R**	
pimple	—grano	rash	—salpullido
pin	—alfiler	recovery room	—sala de recuperación
placenta, afterbirth	—placenta	rectum	—recto
plague, epidemic	—peste, epidemia, plaga	relatives, relations	—parientes
planned parenthood	—paternidad responsable	release from the hospital, to consider cured	—dar de alta
pneumonia	—pulmonía	remain silent or quiet	—guardar silencio, callarse
poisoning	—envenenamiento, emponzoñamiento, intoxicación	remedy	—medicina, medicamento, remedio
policy	—política, póliza	remove stitches	—quitar puntos
polio, poliomyelitis	—poliomielitis, parálisis infantil	repair (tissues)	—reparar (tejidos)
porcelain	—porcelana	respiration, respiratory, breathing	—respiración, respiratorio
portable washbasin or washbowl	—palangana	Rh factor	—factor Rh
postpartum "blues"	—depresión del sobreparto (postparto)	rheumatic fever	—fiebre reumática
		rhythm method (contraceptive)	—método(anticonceptivo) del ritmo
postpartum hemorrhage	—hemorragia del sobreparto	rib	—costilla
postpartum, post-delivery	—sobreparto, puerperio	right auricle	—aurícula derecha
		ringworm	—tiña, culebrilla
potassium	—potasio	root	—raíz
pregnancy	—embarazo, estado de gestación	rubber bandage	—venda o vendaje de goma
pregnancy cycle	—ciclo gravídico		
pregnancy test	—prueba de embarazo	**S**	
pregnant	—embarazada, encinta	safety pin	—imperdible

safety razor	—máquina de afeitar	sprain	—torcedura, distensión
sanity	—juicio sano, cordura	state of pregnancy	—estado de gravidez, preñez, estado de gestación, embarazo
scab	—costra		
scale	—báscula		
scalpel, surgical knife	—escalpelo, bisturí	stay in bed	—guardar cama
scar	—cicatriz	sterile or sterilized cloths	—paños esterilizados
schizophrenia	—esquizofrenia	sternum	—esternón
Sciatic neuritis	—neuritis ciática	stethoscope	—estetoscopio
scissors	—tijeras	stick out one's tongue	—sacar la lengua
sclerotic	—esclerótico		
sedative for sleep	—sedante para dormir	stiff neck, torticollis	—dolor de cuello, tortícolis
semen	—esperma	stimulant	—estimulante
senile dementia	—demencia senil	sting or bite, as of an insect	—picadura
set of teeth	—dentadura		
seven-month baby	—sietemesino(a)	stitches, sutures	—puntos, suturas
sexual relations, sexual intercourse	—relaciones sexuales	stomach	—estómago
sharp pain	—dolor agudo	stomach ache	—dolor de estómago
sheets, bedsheets	—sábanas	straitjacket (straightjacket)	—camisa de fuerza
shin of the leg, blackhead	—espinilla	stretcher	—camilla
shock	—choque, shock	stroke	—apoplejía, derrame, golpe de cerebro
sickness, illness	—enfermedad, mal	stutterer	—tartamudo(a)
silver	—plata	suffocation	—sofocacion, asfixia, ahogo
sinusitis, sinus trouble	—sinusitis	sugar	—azúcar
sleep	—dormir, sueño	suicide	—suicidio
sleep-inducing drug, soporific	—soporífero	sunburn	—quemadura del sol
slit	—cortadura, corte, cortada	sunburn lotion	—loción contra la quemadura del sol
slumped shoulders	—hombros encorvados, cargado(a) de espaldas	sunstroke, heatstroke	—insolación
		suntan lotion	—loción para broncear
small intestine	—intestino delgado	supervisor	—supervisor(a)
smallpox	—viruela	surgeon	—médico(a), cirujano(a)
smear	—unto, untar	surgery	—cirugía, operación quirúrgica
soap	—jabón		
social security	—seguro social, seguridad social	surgery room	—sala de cirugía
sodium	—sodio	surgical knife, scalpel	—escalpelo, bisturí
solvent	—solvente	surgical operation	—operación quirúrgica, cirugía
soporific, sleep-inducing drug	—soporífero	swallowed objects	—objetos tragados
sore muscle	—músculo doloroso	sweat, perspiration	—sudor, transpiración
sound, probe	—sonda	swelled, swollen	—hinchado(a)
spasm	—espasmo	swelling	—hinchazón
specialist	—especialista	swollen tonsils	—amígdalas inflamadas
spell of fainting, fainting fit	—desmayo	symptom	—síntoma
spermatozoan	—espermatozoide	syphylis	—sífilis
spinal column, spine, backbone	—espina dorsal, espinazo, columna vertebral	syringe, hypodermic needle	—jeringa, jeringuilla
spit, sputum	—esputo	**T**	
spittoon	—escupidero	take (someone's) pulse	—tomar el pulso
spleen	—bazo	TB	—tuberculosis, tisis
splint, to put on a splint	—tablilla, entablillar	tear duct	—conducto lacrimal
splinters	—astillas	teaspoonful	—cucharadita
spoonful	—cucharada	technician	—técnico(a)
		temperature	—temperatura, fiebre
		temple	—sien

testicles	—testículos
testosterone	—testosterona
test tube	—tubo de ensayo
tetanus	—tétano
therapy	—terapia
thermometer	—termómetro
thigh	—muslo
thin, slender	—delgado(a)
thread	—hilo
three times a day	—tres veces al día
throat	—garganta
tissue	—tejido
toes, fingers	—dedos del pie, dedos de la mano
tongue	—lengua
tonic	—tónico
tonsils	—amígdalas
toothache	—dolor de muela, de diente
toothbrush	—cepillo de dientes
toothpaste	—pasta de dientes, crema dental
total anesthesia	—anestesia total
toxemia	—toxemia
transfusion	—transfusión
trauma	—trauma, traumatismo
treatment	—tratamiento
tremor	—temblor
triceps muscle	—músculo triceps
triplets	—trillizos(as)
trouble	—afección, achaque, dificultad, inconveniente
tubal ligation	—ligadura de trompas
tweezers	—pinzas
twins	—mellizos(as), gemelos(as)
twisted or pulled muscle	—músculo torcido
twisted neck	—cuello torcido
tube	—tubo
tuberculosis, TB	—tuberculosis, tisis
tumor	—tumor
turpentine	—aguarrás, trementina
typhoid fever	—fiebre tifoidea

U

ulcer	—úlcera
unconsciousness	—falta de conocimiento
underwriters	—aseguradores
unguent, salve	—ungüento, pomada
unnecesary noise	—ruido o bulla innecesaria
unrefined food	—alimento sin refinar
upset	—trastorno, trastornar
urgency	—urgencia
urgent	—urgente
urinalysis	—análisis de orina, urinálisis
urinate	—orinar
urine	—orina
uterine cavity	—cavidad uterina

uterus	—útero
uvula	—úvula o campanilla

V

vaccination	—vacunación
vaccine	—vacuna
vagina	—vagina
vaginal douche	—ducha vaginal
vaginal flow or secretion	—flujo vaginal
vaginal tablets (contraceptive)	—pastillas o tabletas anticonceptivas vaginales
vaginitis	—vaginitis
valve	—válvula
varicose veins	—várices
vasectomy	—vasectomía
vaseline	—vaselina
vein	—vena
venereal	—venéreo
ventricle	—ventrículo
ventricular cavity	—cavidad del ventrículo
vertebra	—vértebra
veterinarian, veterinary	—veterinario
virus	—virus
visual defect	—defecto de la vista
vitamin	—vitamina
voluntary agencies	—agencias voluntarias
vomit, vomiting	—vómito

W

waist	—cintura
waiting room	—sala de espera
wakefulness	—desvelo
walker	—andador
wants	—deseos
waters, bag of	—bolsa de aguas, bolsa amniótica
weak	—débil
weight at birth	—peso al nacer
wheel chair	—silla de ruedas
whole grain bread	—pan integral
wipe on, daub, smear	—untar
wound	—herida
wrist, carpus	—muñeca, carpo o huesos de la muñeca

X

X-ray photograph	—radiografía
X-rays	—rayos X (equis)

Y

yellow fever	—fiebre amarilla

Z

zinc oxide ointment	—pomada o ungüento de óxido de zinc

VOCABULARIO GENERAL

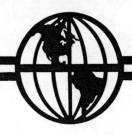

abierto(a)	—open
abrir	—to open
absoluto(a)	—absolute
abuelo(a)	—grandfather, grandmother
abuelos(as)	—grandparents
aburrido(a)	—bored
acá, aquí	—here
aceptante	—acceptor
acercarse	—to draw near, to approach
acomodar	—to accommodate, adapt
aconsejar	—to advise, give advice
acordarse, recordar	—to remember, recall
acostarse	—to go to bed
acostumbrarse	—to become accustomed
achaque habitual o cronico	—sickliness, habitual or cronic ailment
actualidad	—now, the present time
adelgazar	—to reduce, get or become thinner
además	—besides
administrar	—to administer
admisiones	—admissions
¿adónde?	— where?, where to?
aeromoza, azafata	—stewardess, airline hostess
aeropuerto	—airport
afeitarse	—to shave
aficionado(a)	—amateur, fan
agilidad	—agility
agonía	—anguish, death pangs
agotarse	—overdo, become exhausted
agua	—water
agua hervida	—boiled water
aguja	—needle
ahijado(a)	—godson, goddaughter
ahora	—now
ahora mismo	—right now, right away
aire puro	—pure air
a la derecha	—to your (the) right
a la izquierda	—to your (the) left
alarmar	—to alarm
alcoba	—bedroom
alegría	—happiness, joy
al fin y al cabo	—finally, in the final analysis
alguna vez	—sometime
algunas veces	—sometimes, at times

alimento	—item of food
allá, allí	—there
alma	—soul
almuerzo	—lunch
alquilar	—to rent, hire
alto(a)	—high, tall
alumno(a)	—student
amanecer	—to dawn, start the day
amar	—to love
amarillo(a)	—yellow
amigo(a)	—friend, boy friend, girl friend,
amor	—love
amputar	—to amputate
ancho(a)	—wide, broad
andamio	—scaffold, suspended walkway
angustia	—anguish, anxiety
animar	—to cheer up, infuse optimism
ánimo	—optimism, energy, spirit
anochecer	—evening, dusk, to grow dark
antes de	—before
año	—year
año bisiesto	—leap year
Año Nuevo	—New Year
apellido	—last or family name
apenas	—just about, scarcely, hardly
aplaudir	—to applaud
aprovechar	—to take advantage of, benefit from
árbol	—tree
arrendar	—to rent, rent out
artritis	—arthritis
ascendencia	—ancestry
asustarse	—to become frightened
atender	—to take care of, attend to, pay attention to
atractivo(a)	—attractive
a través	—through
atropellar	—to run over, knock down
aunque	—although
automóvil	—car
avanzar	—to advance

a veces	—sometimes, at times	cartas personales	—personal letters
avenida	—avenue	carteles	—posters
¡Ay!	—Ouch!, Oh!	casarse	—to get married
ayudar	—to help	casero(a)	—homemade
azafata, aeromoza	—stewardess, airline hostess	casi	—almost
		cena	—supper
azul	—blue	cerrado(a)	—closed
		charlar	—to chat
B		chancro	—chancre
		chocar	—to collide, to crash, shock
baile	—dance		
bajar	—to go down, lower, sink	clase	—kind, class
		cobija	—blanket
banco	—bank, bench	cobrar	—to charge, collect (money)
bañarse	—to take a bath, bathe		
		cocina	—kitchen
baño, cuarto de baño	—bath, bathroom	colonia	—district, colony
barato(a)	—cheap	comedor	—dining room
baúl	—trunk	¿cómo?	—how?, what?
beber	—to drink	cómodo(a)	—comfortable, convenient
belleza	—beauty		
benéfico(a), beneficioso(a), provechoso(a)	—beneficial, profitable	compañero(a)	—companion
		compañero(a) de cuarto	—roommate
besar	—to kiss		
biberón	—baby bottle	comprar	—to buy
biología	—biology	compromiso	—commitment, appointment, obligation
blanco(a)	—white		
bonito(a)	—pretty, cute		
boleto	—ticket	conferencia	—conference, lecture, meeting
botón	—button		
buscar	—to look for, seek	conocer	—to know, be acquainted with, meet
C		conseguir	—to get, obtain, succeed in
caer, caerse	—to fall, to fall down	consejo	—advice, counsel
		consignador	—consignor
café	—coffee	consignatario	—consignee
café, marrón	—brown	consumir	—to consume, to eat
calcetines	—socks	contar con	—to rely on, have available, count on
callejón	—alley		
calor, caliente	—heat, hot	contestación	—reply, answer
calzar	—to shoe, englove, block, wedge, fill teeth	contrario(a)	—opposite, contrary
		correo(s)	—post office, mail
cambiar dinero	—to change or convert money	compartir	—to share
		construir	—to build, construct
camioneta	—station wagon	cuaderno	—notebook
campaña	—campaign	cuadra, manzana	—city block, whole city block
campesino(a)	—peasant, country dweller		
		cuadro	—blackboard, picture, switchboard
capaz, hábil	—able, capable		
caramelos, dulces	—candy, pieces of candy	¿cual?	—which?, which one?
		¿cuándo?	—when?
carne de borrego o cordero	—lamb meat	¿cuánto(a)?, ¿cuántos(as)?	—how much?, how many?
carne de conejo	—rabbit meat	cubrir	—to cover
carne de guajolote o pavo	—turkey meat	cuidar a, de	—to take care of
carne de pato	—duck meat	cumpleaños	—birthday
carne de puerco	—pig meat, pork	cumplir	—to fulfill, to discharge, to perform, to carry out
carne de ternero	—calf meat, veal		
carne de vaca	—bovine meat, beef		
caro(a)	—expensive		
carretera	—highway	cuñado(a)	—brother-in-law, sister-in-law

D

darse prisa	—to hurry
defectuoso(a)	—defective
dejar, salir	—to leave
dejar de, parar	—to stop
deleitarse	—to enjoy, take delight
de ningún modo	—in no way
depender	—to depend
deportes marítimos	—ocean sports
derecho	—right (under law)
derecho(a)	—right (location)
derecho, directo	—straight ahead
derecho(a), recto(a)	—straight, unswerving
desarrollo	—development
desayunar	—to eat breakfast
descansar	—to rest
descuidar	—to neglect, be careless
desear	—to want, desire
desempeñar	—to fulfill, carry out, perform
desinfectar	—to disinfect
despensa	—storeroom, pantry
despertador	—alarm clock
despertarse	—to wake up
detalles, pormenores	—details
día de fiesta, día feriado	—holiday
Día de Navidad	—Christmas Day
dieta equilibrada	—balanced diet
dieta sin sal	—salt-free diet
difícil	—hard, difficult
dinero	—money
diploma	—diploma
diversos(as)	—several, various, diverse
¿dónde?	—where?
dormitorio	—dormitory, bedroom
ducha	—shower
dueño(a)	—owner
durante	—during
durar	—to last

E

editorial	—editorial
educación física	—physical education
educado(a)	—raised, brought up, well-mannered, educated
efectivo(a)	—real, effective
el, la, los, las	—the
embromar	—to tease, annoy, play jokes on, harm
emparentarse	—to become related
empeorar	—to make worse, worsen
en cambio	—on the other hand
endorsante	—endorser
engañar	—to deceive, fool
enrojecer(se)	—to redden, blush, turn red

en seguida	—right away
enseñar	—to teach, show
entidad	—institution, (corporate) entity
entonces	—then
entrada	—ticket (to the theater, etc.), entrance
enviar	—to send
equivocarse	—to make a mistake, to err, be wrong
escarcha	—frost
escritorio	—office, desk
escuchar	—to listen
escuchar (el programa)	—to listen to (the program)
espectador(a)	—spectator
esperar	—to wait, wait for, hope, expect
espléndido(a)	—splendid
esposo(a)	—husband, wife, spouse
esquina	—corner
estar	—to be
este, oriente	—east
estrecho(a)	—narrow
estrenar	—to wear or show for the first time
exagerar	—to exaggerate, overdo
excelente	—excellent
explicar	—to explain
expuesto(a)	—exposed, vulnerable
extranjero(a)	—foreigner

F

fácil	—easy
factura	—invoice, bill
fallecido(a)	—deceased
faltarle a uno dinero	—to lack or need money
favorito(a)	—favorite, pet
felicitar	—to congratulate
figurarse, imaginarse	—to imagine
flan	—pudding
fotografía, foto	—photography, photo, (photographed) picture
frasco	—flask, bottle, jar
frecuentemente	—frequently
frío(a)	—cool, cold
fruta	—fruit
fuerte	—strong
fumar	—to smoke
función	—function
funcionar	—to function

G

galletas	—cookies, crackers
ganar	—to earn, win
garaje	—garage
gerente(a)	—manager
gozar de	—to enjoy

gran mortandad	—decimation	joven	—young, youth
grande	—big, large	joyas	—jewels
gris	—gray (grey)	juramento de	—Hippocratic
gritar	—to shout, cry out	Hipócrates	oath
guardar	—to keep, retain, put away, hold		
guardián	—guardian	**L**	
gustar	—to like, please, be pleasing to	lado	—side
		ladrón(a)	—thief
gusto	—taste, pleasure	lágrima	—tear (of the eye)
		la hora de	
H		acostarse	—bedtime
		lápiz	—pencil
hablar	—to speak, talk	las afueras	—the outskirts, suburbs
hacer	—to do, make	lastimarse	—to hurt oneself, be
hacia	—toward		injured or hurt
hambre	—hunger	lavarse	—to wash oneself, to
hay	—there is, there are		wash up, to get washed
hembra	—female	leche en polvo	—dry milk, powdered
hereditario(a)	—hereditary		milk
herir, herirse	—to wound, to get wounded	leche malteada	—malted milk
		leer	—to read
hermano(a) adoptivo(a)	—adopted brother, sister	legumbres, verduras, vegetales	—vegetables
hermoso(a)	—good-looking, beautiful, handsome	lejos	—far, far away, distant(ly)
hijo(a)	—son, daughter	lento(a),	
hogar	—home, hearth	lentamente	—slow, slowly
hombre	—man	levantarse	—to get up, get out
honor	—honor		of bed
hospedarse	—to lodge, be lodged	libertad	—freedom, liberty
I		libro	—book
		limonada	—lemonade
iglesia	—church	limpiar	—to clean, cleanse
impaciente	—impatient	limpio(a)	—clean
impedir	—to prevent, keep from, impede	listo(a)	—ready, smart
		llamar	—to call
importante	—important	llegar	—to arrive
incapacitado(a)	—incapacitated	lleno(a)	—full
inconsciente	—unconscious	llevar	—to take, carry
indudablemente	—undoubtedly	loción	—lotion
infeliz	—unhappy, poor soul, unfortunate	lugar	—place
		luna	—moon
información	—information	luz roja	—red light
insignificante	—insignificant		
insistir en	—to insist on	**M**	
instrucciones	—instructions, directions	madrastra	—stepmother
instruir	—educate, instruct	madre	—mother
inteligente	—intelligent	madrina	—godmother
inteligente	—intelligent	maestro(a)	—teacher, masculine
intenciones	—intentions, purposes		and feminine
intentar	—to try to, to attempt	malgastar	—to squander, spend
invitar	—to invite		unwisely
ir	—to go	malo(a)	—bad
irse	—to go away, leave	manar	—to pour forth, flow
isla	—island	mandar	—order, command,
itinerario	—itinerary, routing, schedule of travel		send
izquierdo(a)	—left (location)	manta, frazada	—blanket
jalea	—jelly	mantenerse	—to keep, stay or
jardín	—garden		maintain oneself,
jefe de familia	—head of the family		be maintained

mantequilla	—butter	ocupado(a)	—busy, occupied
manzana, cuadra	—whole city block, city block	oeste	—west
		ofrecer	—to offer
maravilloso(a)	—wonderful, marvellous	oír	—to hear, to listen
masculino(a)	—masculine, male	ojalá	—I, you, etc., wish that
matemáticas	—mathematics, math		
mayor	—older, larger	oler	—to smell, to give off an odor
medio(a) hermano(a)	—half brother, half sister	olvidar(se)	—to forget, be forgetful
medir	—to measure	ordenar	—to order, command, ordain
mejorar	—to improve, get better		
memoria	—memory		
menor	—younger, smaller	**P**	
mensual	—monthly		
menú	—menu	padecer	—to suffer (an illness, etc.)
merecer	—to deserve, merit		
mermelada	—marmelade	padrastro	—stepfather
mes	—month	padre	—father
mesa	—table	padrino	—godfather
meter	—to insert, put in	pagar	—to pay
método	—method	país	—country
miedo	—fear	palabra	—word
mientras	—while	pan	—bread
mirar	—to look at	papel	—paper, role
moda	—fashion	pared	—wall
modelo	—model	parque	—park
momento	—moment	partido	—game, political party
moneda	—coin		
montón	—pile	pasaporte	—passport
morir	—to die	pasar	—to pass, pass by, happen
muchacho(a)	—boy, girl		
muchísimo(a), muchísimos(as)	—very much, very many	paz	—peace
		peinarse	—to comb one's hair
muelas	—(back) teeth		
muerte	—death	película	—film
mujer	—woman, wife	peligroso	—dangerous, hazardous
		pellizcar	—to pinch
N		peluquero(a)	—barber, hairdresser
		pena, pesar	—sorrow, pity, embarrassment
nacer	—to be born		
naturaleza	—nature	pensar	—to think, to intend
naturalidad	—naturalness	pequeño(a)	—little, small
Navidad	—Christmas	perder	—to lose
necesidad	—necessity, need	perfume	—perfume
necesitado(a)	—needed, needy	perjudicar	—to damage, harm, hurt
negarse	—to refuse	permiso	—permission, license
negativo(a)	—negative	pero	—but
negro(a)	—black	pesado(a)	—heavy
ninguna parte	—nowhere	pesar	—to weigh
niño(a)	—baby, small child	pescador(a)	—fisherman, fisherwoman
nitrógeno	—nitrogen		
noche	—night	piso	—floor, apartment
Nochebuena	—Christmas Eve	pinchar	—to pierce, puncture, stick
norte	—north		
novio(a)	—boyfriend, girlfriend, "steady date"	pizarra	—blackboard, slate
		plato	—plate, dish
nueces	—nuts	pluma	—pen, feather
nuera	—daughter-in-law	pobre	—poor, unfortunate
nuevo(a)	—new	pobreza	—poverty
		poder	—to be able, can
O		póliza de seguros	—insurance policy
		porcentaje	—percentage
obrero	—workman,		

por ciento	—per cent	regalo	—present, gift
por día	—per diem, per day, by the day	regañar	—to scold
		regatear	—to bargain, argue over price
pormenores, detalles	—details		
posible	—possible	remover	—to stir, stir up, move around
positivo(a)	—positive		
postizo(a)	—false, artificial	repetir	—to repeat
postre	—dessert	reservado(a)	—reserved
precaución	—precaution, care	respirar	—to breathe
preferir	—to prefer	respuesta	—response, answer, reply
pregunta	—question		
preocuparse	—to worry, be concerned	restaurante	—restaurant
		resultado	—result, outcome
presenciar	—to witness	resultar	—to turn out, to result
presentar	—to introduce, present		
prestar	—to lend, give	retrato	—picture, portrait
primo(a)	—cousin	reunión	—meeting
probabilidad	—probability	revista	—magazine
propina	—tip	riqueza	—wealth
propósitos	—purposes, intentions	rojo(a)	—red
provechoso(a), benéfico(a)	—profitable, beneficial	romper	—to break, tear, rip
		ropa	—clothes, clothing
próximo(a)	—next	ropa de invierno	—winter clothing
publicidad	—publicity, advertising	ropa interior	—underwear
		rutina, rutinario(a)	—routine
pudín	—pudding		
pueblo	—people, town		
puerta	—door, gate		

Q

		S	
¿qué?	—what?, which?	sábana	—sheet
quebrar	—to break	saber	—to know
quedarse	—to stay, remain, be	sabroso(a)	—delightful, delicious
quedarse con	—to keep	sacar	—to take out, remove, withdraw
quejarse	—to complain		
querer	—to want, wish, love, have affection for	sala	—living room
		sala-comedor	—living room with dining area
¿quién?, ¿a quién?	—who?, whom?	sala familiar	—family room
química	—chemistry	salir	—to leave, go out
quiste	—cyst	salir de vacaciones	—to take a, go on, leave on, vacation
quitar	—to remove, take out, off or away from		
		salvo	—except
		sed	—thirst

R

		semáforo	—traffic light
		semana	—week
rama	—branch, division	sencillo(a)	—simple, single
rancho	—ranch	sentarse	—to sit down
rápidamente	—fast, quickly, rapidly, speedily	sentirse	—to feel
		señor, señora, señorita	—Mr., Mrs., Miss
rapidez	—rapidity, speed, quickness	separar	—to separate
		ser	—to be
rebajar	—to reduce, lessen, diminish	ser gordo(a) u obeso(a)	—to be overweight, fat, obese
		servilleta	—napkin
rebajar de peso	—to reduce, lose weight	siempre	—always
recetar	—to prescribe	sífilis	—syphilis
recoger	—to pick up, gather	siglo	—century
recomendar	—recommend	silencio	—silence
reconstruir	—to reconstruct, rebuild, remodel	silla	—chair
		simpático(a)	—nice, pleasant, congenial, engaging, amusing
recuperar	—to recuperate, recover		
regalar	—to give away, give		

sin	—without
sirena	—siren
sobre todo	—above all
sobrino(a)	—nephew, niece
sociedad	—society
soda gaseosa	—soda pop, soft drink
sol	—sun
solo(a)	—alone, lonely
sólo, solamente	—only
sombra	—shade, shadow
sonreír	—to smile
sopa	—soup
sorpresa	—surprise
suceder	—to happen
suegro(a)	—father-in-law, mother-in-law
sueño equilibrado	—even, peaceful sleep
suficiente	—enough, sufficient
sufrir	—to suffer
sugerir	—to suggest
suprimir	—to extirpate, remove, suppress
sur	—south

T

también	—also
tanto(a), tantos(as)	—as or so much, as or so many
tardar en	—to be long in(doing something)
tarde	—late, afternoon
tarjetas de Navidad	—Christmas cards
taza	—cup
té	—tea
temporada	—time, season, period
temprano	—early
tenedor	—fork
tener	—to have
tener que	—to have to
tener años	—to be years old
tener cuidado	—to be careful
tener exceso de peso	—to be overweight
tener éxito	—to be successful
tener lugar	—to take place
tener miedo	—to be afraid
tener vergüenza	—to be ashamed
tenga la bondad	—please
terminar	—to finish, end
tetera	—nipple on a baby's bottle
tienda, almacén	—store
tío(a)	—uncle, aunt
todavía	—still, yet
tomar	—to take, eat or drink
tomar nota	—to note down
tonto(a)	—fool, foolish
torero	—bullfighter
tortilla	—tortilla, omelet
trabajar	—to work
trabajoso(a)	—hard, difficult, requiring effort
traducir	—to translate

traer	—to bring
traje	—suit
tranquilo(a)	—tranquil, calm
transportar	—to transport
tratar	—to treat, to deal with socially
tratar de	—to try to, to attempt
tren	—train
triste	—sad
tristeza	—sadness
turista	—tourist
turno, cita	—turn, appointment

U

último modelo	—latest model
un, una, unos, unas	—a, an, some
uniforme	—uniform
universidad	—university
universitario(a)	—of a university, university student

V

valer	—to be worth
variar	—to vary
varón	—male
varonil	—male, masculine
vaso	—glass
vecino(a)	—neighbor
vegetariano(a)	—vegetarian
vehículo	—vehicle
vejez	—old age
veloz	—fast, speedy
vencimiento	—act of becoming or falling due
vender	—to sell
venida	—coming, arrival
ventana	—window
ver	—to see
verdadero(a)	—true
verde	—green
vestido	—woman's dress
vestirse	—to get dressed
viajar	—to travel
viaje	—trip, voyage
viajero(a)	—traveler
vida	—life
viejo(a)	—old, old man or woman
visita	—visit, visitor
vivir	—to live
voluntario(a)	—volunteer
vuelo	—flight
vulnerable, expuesto(a)	—vulnerable, exposed

Y

ya que	—since
yerno	—son-in-law

Z

zapato	—shoe

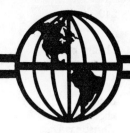

A

a, an, some —un, una, unos, unas
above all —sobre todo
absolute —absoluto(a)
able, capable —hábil, capaz
acceptor —aceptante
accommodate —acomodar, servir
act of becoming
  or falling due —vencimiento
admissions —admisiones
adolescent, teen-ager —adolescente
adopted brother, sister —hermano(a) adoptivo(a)
administer —administrar
advance —avanzar
advertising —publicidad, propaganda
advise —aconsejar
afraid —miedoso, teniendo
  miedo
after —después
agility —agilidad
agony —agonía, dolor intenso
airline hostess,
  stewardess —azafata, aeromoza
airport —aeropuerto
alarm —alarma
alarm clock —despertador
although —aunque
amateur, fan —aficionado(a)
amusing —simpático, divertido
ancestry —ascendencia
anguish —angustia, agonía
applaud —aplaudir
appointment —cita, compromiso,
  turno
as or so much, as —tanto(a),
  or so many tantos(as)
ashamed —avergonzado(a)
at least —por lo menos
attempt —intentar, tratar de
attractive —atractivo(a),
  llamativo(a)
aunt —tía
avenue —avenida

B

baby —niño(a), bebé,
  criatura, recién nacido
balanced diet —dieta equilibrada
bank, bench —banco
bathroom —baño, cuarto de baño
beauty —belleza
beautiful —hermoso(a), bello(a)

become accustomed —acostumbrarse
become inflamed —inflamarse
become related —emparentarse
bed —cama
bedroom —alcoba, dormitorio
bedtime —hora de acostarse
beneficial, profitable —benéfico(a),
  provechoso(a)
be overweight, fat —tener exceso de peso,
  obese ser gordo(a) u obeso(a)
besides —además
biology —biología
black —negro(a)
blackboard —pizarrón, cuadro
blanket —manta, cobija, frazada
blue —azul
body —cuerpo
boiled water —agua hervida
book —libro
bored —aburrido(a)
bottle, flask —botella, frasco
boy —muchacho
boyfriend —amigo, novio
branch —rama
break —quebrar, romper
breakfast —desayuno
breathe —respirar
bring —traer
bring up, raise —educar, criar
brother —hermano
brother-in-law —cuñado
brown —café, marrón
build —construir
busy —ocupado(a)
butter —mantequilla
button —botón

C

call —llamar
campaign —campaña
candy —caramelos, dulces
capable, able —capaz, hábil
capital —capital
car —carro
careful —cuidadoso(a)
carry —llevar
carry out —desempeñar,
  cumplir, llevar a
  cabo
century —siglo
chair —silla
chalk —tiza, gis

change money	—cambiar dinero	development	—desarrollo
charge money	—cobrar dinero	dew	—rocío
chat	—charlar	die	—morir
cheap	—barato(a), económico(a)	diet	—alimentacion, régimen alinmenticio
cheer up	—animar(se), alegrar(se)		
chocolate	—chocolate	direct	—directo(a)
Christmas Day	—Día de Navidad	discharge	—cumplir, desempeñar, cesantear
Christmas Eve	—Nochebuena		
church	—iglesia	disinfect	—desinfectar
city block	—cuadra, manzana	district	—distrito, colonia
clean	—limpio(a)	diverse, various,	
clothes	—ropa	several	—diverso(a)
coffee	—café	division	—rama, división
coin	—moneda	door	—puerta
colony	—colonia, distrito	dormitory	—dormitorio, residencia estudiantil
collect money	—cobrar dinero		
collide	—chocar	draw near, approach	—acercarse, aproximarse, arrimarse
collision	—colisión, choque, encuentro		
comb	—peinar, peine	drink	—beber, tomar
comb one's hair	—peinarse	dry milk	—leche en polvo
comfortable,		during	—durante
convenient	—cómodo(a)		
command	—ordenar, mandar		
companion	—compañero(a)	**E**	
complain	—quejarse		
conference	—conferencia, congreso	earn	—ganar
congenial	—simpático(a)	easy	—fácil
congratulate	—felicitar	east	—este, oriente
consignee	—consignatario(a)	eat	—comer, tomar
consignor	—consignador(a)	editorial	—editorial
consume	—consumir	educate, raise, bring up	—instruir, educar, criar
cool, cold	—frío(a)		
corner	—esquina, rincón	educated, raised,	—instruido(a),
corresponding	—correspondiente	brought up	educado(a), criado(a)
cousin	—primo(a)		
cover	—cubrir, tapar	effective	—efectivo(a)
cute	—bonito(a), mono(a)	enforce	—obligar o cumplir
		engaging	—simpático
		enjoy	—deleitarse, disfrutar, gozar de
D			
		enough	—suficiente, bastante
dance	—baile	evening, dusk	—anochecer, ocaso
dangerous	—peligroso(a)	even, peaceful	
dare	—atreverse, osar	sleep	—sueño equilibrado
daughter	—hija	exaggerate	—exagerar
daughter-in-law	—nuera	examination	—examen
dawn	—amanecer, salida del sol	excellent	—excelente
		except	—salvo
death pangs, anguish	—agonía, angustia	expect	—esperar
deceased	—fallecido(a)	explain	—explicar
deceive	—engañar	exposed	—expuesto(a), vulnerable
defective	—defectuoso(a)		
definition	—definición	extirpate, remove	—extirpar, suprimir
delightful, delicious	—sabroso(a), delicioso(a)		
depend on	—depender de, contar con	**F**	
depressed	—deprimido(a)	false	—postizo(a), falso(a)
depressing	—deprimente	fall, fall down	—caer, caerse
depressive	—depresivo(a)	family	—familia
deserve	—merecer, ameritar	far	—lejos, distante, alejado(a)
dessert	—postre	fast	—rápidamente, velozmente
details	—detalles, pormenores		

father	—padre	insincerity	—doblez
father-in-law	—suegro	insist on	—insistir en
felt	—sentido	instituciones	—entidades, instituciones
female	—hembra		
feminine	—femenino(a)	instructions	—instrucciones
film	—película	insurance	—seguro
flight	—vuelo	intelligent	—inteligente
floor	—piso	intentions	—intenciones, propósitos
fool	—tonto(a), bobo(a)	introduce	—presentar, introducir
fork	—tenedor	invalid policy	—póliza o política inválida
frequently	—frecuentemente, a menudo		
fulfill	—desempeñar, cumplir	invoice	—factura
full	—lleno(a), repleto(a)	island	—isla
function	—función	itinerary	—itinerario
		I, you, he, etc., wish that	—ojalá que

G

garage	—garaje	
get	—conseguir, obtener	**J**
get dressed	—vestirse	
get ready	—preparar(se)	just about
get sick	—enfermarse	
girl	—muchacha, niña, chica	

girlfriend	—novia, amiga
give advice	—aconsejar

just about	—apenas, más o menos, unos(as), alrededor de

K

keep	—mantener(se), guardar, quedarse con
glass	—vaso, vidrio
go	—ir
goddaughter	—ahijada
godfather	—padrino
godmother	—madrina
go down	—bajar, amainar, disminuir, menguar

kiss	—besar
kitchen	—cocina
knife	—cuchillo
know	—conocer, saber

godson	—ahijado
good	—bueno(a)
good-looking	—hermoso(a)
go on vacation	—salir de vacaciones
go to bed	—acostarse
go out	—salir
grandparents	—abuelos
green	—verde

L

lack money	—faltarle a uno dinero
lamb	—cordero
larger	—mayor, más grande
last	—durar, permanecer
last or family name	—apellido
leap year	—año bisiesto

H

handsome	—hermoso, buen mozo
happen	—suceder, pasar
hardly, scarcely	—apenas
hard-working	—trabajador(a)
hazardous	—peligroso(a)
healthy	—saludable, sano(a)
heat	—calor
highway	—carretera, calzada
holiday	—día de fiesta, día feriado

leave	—dejar, salir, irse
leave on vacation	—salir de vacaciones
lecture	—conferencia
life	—vida
life insurance	—seguro de vida
listen to (the program)	—escuchar (el programa)
living room	—sala
living room with dining area	—sala-comedor
look (at)	—mirar
lotion	—loción
lunch	—almuerzo, almorzar

hollow needle	—aguja hueca
hope	—esperar, esperanza
how?	—¿cómo?

I

M

magazine	—revista
maintain, keep oneself	—mantenerse
make worse	—empeorar
male	—varón, varonil, masculino(a)

imagine	—figurarse, imaginarse
impatient	—impaciente
incapacitated	—incapacitado(a)

malted milk	—leche malteada

man	—hombre
manager	—gerente
masculine	—masculino(a), varonil
mathematics, math	—matemáticas
measure	—medir, medida
meat	—carne
memory	—memoria, recuerdo
menu	—menú
method	—método
model	—modelo
moment	—momento
money	—dinero
month	—mes
monthly	—mensual
moon	—luna
mother	—madre
mother-in-law	—suegra
Mr., Mrs., Miss	—señor, señora, señorita

N

narrow	—estrecho(a), angosto(a)
naturally	—naturalmente
nature	—naturaleza
near	—cerca (de), cercano(a)
necessity, need	—necesidad
neglect	—descuidar, descuido
neighbor	—vecino(a)
nephew	—sobrino
new	—nuevo(a)
New Year	—Año Nuevo
nice	—simpático(a), agradable
night	—noche
north	—norte
notebook	—cuaderno
note down	—tomar nota o apunte, anotar, apuntar
now	—ahora, la actualidad, actualmente, ya
nowhere	—ninguna parte
nuts	—nueces

O

obtain	—obtener, conseguir
ocean sports	—deportes marítimos
offer	—ofrecer
office	—oficina, despacho, escritorio
old	—viejo(a)
old age	—vejez
older	—mayor, más viejo(a)
only	—sólo, solamente, únicamente
open	—abierto(a), abrir
optimism, energy, spirit	—ánimo
order	—ordenar, mandar, pedir
orientation film	—película orientadora
overdo	—agotarse, extremar la nota
owner	—dueño(a), poseedor(a)

P

pantry	—despensa
paper	—papel
pass	—pasar, pase
passport	—pasaporte
pay	—pagar, pago
pen	—pluma, plumafuente, bolígrafo
people	—gente, pueblo, personas
per cent	—por ciento
percentage	—porcentaje
per diem, per day	—por día
perform	—desempeñar, cumplir, realizar
perfume	—perfume
permission	—permiso, venia
personal letters	—cartas personales
photograph, photo	—fotografía, foto
physical education	—educación física
plate	—plato
picture	—cuadro, fotografía, foto, dibujo
pick up	—recoger, ir a buscar
pierce	—pinchar
pile	—montón, pila
pinch	—pellizcar
pleasant	—simpático, agradable
policy	—póliza, política
poor	—pobre
pork	—carne de puerco
positive	—positivo(a)
possible	—posible
poverty	—pobreza
powdered milk	—leche en polvo
precaution	—precaución, prevención
precisely	—precisamente
prefer	—preferir
present time	—la actualidad, tiempo del presente
pretty	—bonito(a)
probability	—probabilidad
profitable, beneficial	—provechoso(a), benéfico(a), beneficioso(a)
psychologic(al)	—sicológico(a)
publicity	—publicidad, propaganda
pudding	—pudín, flan
puncture	—pinchar
pure air	—aire puro
purpose	—propósito, intención

R

raise, bring up	—educar, criar
raised, brought up	—educado(a), criado(a)
ranch	—rancho
read	—leer
real	—real, efectivo(a), verdadero(a)
rebuild	—reconstruir
recommend	—recomendar
reduce	—rebajar de peso

re-enforce	—reforzar, añadir nuevas fuerzas a	smile	—sonreír
regular visit	—visita regular	socks	—calcetines, medias
rely on	—contar con	soda pop	—(soda) gaseosa
remain	—quedarse, permanecer, mantenerse	soft drink	—(soda) gaseosa
		sometime	—alguna vez
remember	—recordar, acordarse de	sometimes	—a veces, algunas veces
remodel	—reconstruir	son	—hijo
remove	—extirpar, suprimir, quitar, sacar	son-in-law	—yerno
		so or as much, so or as many	—tanto(a), tantos(as)
rent	—arrendar, alquilar, alquiler	sorrow	—aflicción, congoja, pena, pesar
repair tissues	—reparar los tejidos	specialist	—especialista
repeat	—repetir	splendid	—espléndido(a), magnífico(a)
reply	—contestar, contestación, responder, respuesta	spoon	—cuchara, cucharita
respond	—responder, contestar	sport	—deporte
rest	—descansar, descanso, reposo	squander	—malgastar, derrochar, despilfarrar
restaurant	—restaurante	stay	—mantenerse, quedarse, permanecer
result	—resultar, resultado		
return	—regreso, vuelta	stephather	—padrastro
right	—derecho(a) (lugar, local), (tener) razón, correcto(a)	stepmother	—madrastra
		stewardess	—aeromoza, azafata
		still	—quieto, callado
right away	—en seguida, ahora mismo	still, yet	—todavía, aún
right (under law)	—derecho	stir, move around	—remover, moverse
room	—cuarto	stop	—dejar de, parar(se), detener(se)
routine	—rutina, rutinario(a)		
routing	—itinerario, plan de rutas o caminos a seguir	store	—tienda, almacén
		storeroom	—despensa, depósito
		straight	—derecho(a), recto(a)
run over, knock down	—atropellar	straight ahead	—derecho, directo
		stranger	—forastero, desconocido
		street	—calle
S		strong	—fuerte
		student	—estudiante
sad	—triste	succed in	—conseguir, lograr
sadness	—tristeza	success	—éxito
salve, unguent	—pomada, ungüento	sufficient	—suficiente
scaffold	—andamio	suffer	—sufrir, padecer
scarcely, hardly	—apenas	suggest	—insinuar, sugerir
schedule of travel	—itinerario	suit	—traje
sell	—vender	supper	—cena
send	—enviar, mandar, expedir, remitir		
separate	—separar	**T**	
several	—diversos(as), varios(as)		
shade, shadow	—sombra	take	—llevar, tomar
shame	—vergüenza, lástima	take a bath	—bañarse
shave	—afeitarse	take advantage of	—aprovechar, aprovecharse de
shower	—ducha, ducharse		
silence	—silencio	take a shower	—ducharse, dare una ducha
simple	—sencillo(a), simple		
since	—ya que, puesto que	take a vacation	—salir de vacaciones
siren	—sirena	take care of	—cuidar a, ocuparse de, atender
sister	—hermana		
sister-in-law	—cuñada	take off	—quitar, retirar
sit down	—sentarse	take out	—sacar, retirar, extraer
sleep	—dormir, sueño		
slow	—lento(a), despacio, despacioso	take place	—tener lugar, suceder, ocurrir
smaller	—menor, más pequeño, más chico	tall, high	—alto(a)
		taste, pleasure	—gusto

teach	—enseñar	**V**	
teacher	—maestro(a), profesor(a)	various	—diversos(as), varios(as)
tease	—embromar, tomar el pelo	veal	—carne de ternero
		vegetables	—vegetales, legumbres, verduras
textbook, text	—libro de texto, texto	vegetarian	—vegetariano
then	—entonces, luego	vehicle	—vehículo
think	—pensar	very much	—muchísimo
through	—a través	visit	—visita
ticket	—boleto, entrada, pasaje	volunteers	—voluntarios
		vulnerable, exposed	—vulnerable, expuesto(a)
time	—tiempo, vez		
tip	—propina	**W**	
to your or the right	—a la derecha		
to your or the left	—a la izquierda	wake up	—despertar(se)
tortilla, omelet	—tortilla	wait, wait for	—esperar
tourist	—turista	want	—querer, deseo, desear
traffic light	—semáforo	wash oneself, wash up, get washed	—lavarse
train	—tren	watch	—contemplar, mirar, reloj
tranquil, calm	—tranquilo(a)		
translate	—traducir	weak	—débil
transport	—transportar, transporte	wealth	—riqueza
travel	—viajar	wear or show for the first time	—estrenar
traveler	—viajero(a)	weigh	—pesar
treat	—tratar	weight	—peso
tree	—árbol	west	—oeste
trip	—viaje	what?	—¿qué?, ¿cómo?
true	—verdad, verdadero(a)	when?	—¿cuándo?
		where?	—¿dónde?
trunk	—baúl	which?	—¿cuál?
try to	—tratar de, intentar, procurar	while	—mientras
		who?, (whom?)	—¿a quién?
turkey	—guajolote, pavo	winter clothing	—ropa de invierno
turn out	—resultar, salir	within	—dentro(de)
		woman's dress	—vestido
U		wonderful, marvelous	—maravilloso(a)
		wound	—herida, herir(se)
uncle	—tío		
underwear	—ropa interior, paños menores	**Y**	
underwriters	—aseguradores	year	—año
undoubtedly	—indudablemente	yellow	—amarillo
ungüent, salve	—ungüento, pomada	young	—joven
university	—universidad	younger	—menor, más joven
university student	—estudiante universitario		

INDEX / INDICE